W9-BDT-104

Sling Training

Big thanks to our families, Stavanger Sports Clinic (location), Jungle Sports (equipment), Gry G. Thorsen (photographer), Lene Løland and Siw Øie Norheim (models), Øyvind and Bent (Norwegian publishers), Anne Mellbye (Mellbye Design), Meg Willett and Susan Bujko (proofreading) and all the experts who contributed with sport specific workouts.

Sling Training

Full Body Suspension Workout

Lennart Krohn-Hansen and Anders Berget

Meyer & Meyer Sport

British Library Cataloguing in Publication Data
A catalogue record for this book is available from the British Library

Sling Training
Maidenhead: Meyer & Meyer Sport (UK) Ltd., 2013
ISBN: 978-1-78255-018-1

1st edition 2013
© 2011 "Jungelboken Forlag AS"

© 2013 by Meyer & Meyer Sport (UK) Ltd.
Aachen, Auckland, Beirut, Budapest, Cairo, Cape Town, Dubai, Hägendorf,
Indianapolis, Maidenhead, Singapore, Sydney, Tehran, Wien

 Member of the World Sport Publishers' Association (WSPA)
www.w-s-p-a.org

Printed by: B.O.S.S Druck und Medien GmbH, Germany
ISBN: 978-1-78255-018-1
E-Mail: info@m-m-sports.com
www.m-m-sports.com

Content

Introduction 8
    Why this book 10
    How did sling training start? 11
    Get started! 12

I   Before You Start 15
    Perfect posture 16
    Core activation 17
    The 80/100 option 17
    Core stability 18
    General tips 19
    Plank core stability 20
    Standing core stability 21
    Sets and repetitions 22
    Rep and set recommendations according to activity 23

II To Work Out in Slings 25
    Basics: backward position 26
    Forward position 28
    Supporting foot 30

III Get the Most Out of the Book 33
    Know your way around 34
    Start position 34
    End position 34
    Sling height 36
    Difficulty level 37

IV Exercises — 39

1 Full Body Workout — 39

1.1	Squat and row	40	1.2	Lunge and fly	41
1.3	Lunge with side bend	42	1.4	One leg squat to lunge	43
1.5	Overhead boxing	44	1.6	Ice skates	45
1.7	Sprinter start	46	1.8	Postural squat	47

2 Lower Body Strength — 49

2.1	One leg squat stand	50	2.2	One leg squat with rotation	51
2.3	Backward lunge	52	2.4	Backward lunge to jump	53
2.5	Stability lunge	54	2.6	One leg deep squat	55
2.7	Hamstring curl	56	2.8	High hamstring curl	57
2.9	One leg hamstring curl	58	2.10	High extension to splits	59
2.11	Sling leg lifts	60	2.12	Inner thigh lifts	61

3 Upper Body Strength — 63

3.1	Kneeling superman	64	3.2	Superman	65
3.3	One hand superman	66	3.4	Flies	67
3.5	Reverse elbow flies	68	3.6	Reverse flies	69
3.7	Y-flies	70	3.8	A-flies	71
3.9	One arm row	72	3.10	Incline pull-ups	73
3.11	Bent arm side press	74	3.12	Side press	75
3.13	External rotation	76	3.14	Internal rotation	77
3.15	Hammer curls	78	3.16	One arm bicep curl	79
3.17	Triceps press	80	3.18	One arm triceps press	81
3.19	Incline push-ups	82	3.20	Push-ups	83
3.21	Push-ups on a fitness ball	83	3.22	Supported dips	84
3.23	Dips	85	3.24	Pull-ups	86
3.25	Incline pull-ups to triceps press				87

4 Core — 89

4.1	Forward lean	90	4.2	Knees off the ground	91
4.3	The plank	92	4.4	Sling cycling	93

4.5	Omega	94	4.6	Sideways omega	95
4.7	Twisted plank	96	4.8	Delta	97
4.9	Body saw	98	4.10	Side plank	99
4.11	Dynamic side plank	100	4.12	Supine plank	101
4.13	One leg supine plank	102	4.14	Supine plank rotation	103
4.15	Sling bridge	104	4.16	Reverse sling cycling	105
4.17	Leg lifts	106	4.18	Wide sling obliques	107

5   Extreme Sling Training **109**

5.1	Extreme plank	110	5.2	Incline handstand press	111
5.3	Handstand press	112	5.4	Twisted side plank	113
5.5	One hand one foot omega	114	5.6	Double poling plank	115
5.7	One arm supported push-up	116	5.8	One arm sling push-ups	116
5.9	Straddle sit to half flair	117	5.10	Wide sling leg lifts	118
5.11	Extreme swing	119	5.12	Hanging leg raises	120
5.13	V-ups	121	5.14	Hanging and turning	122
5.15	Sling handstands	123	5.16	Twisted push-ups	124
5.17	The egg	125	5.18	Hanging sit-ups	126
5.19	Sling squat	127	5.20	Typewriter pull-ups	128
5.21	Supported one hand pull-up				129

6   Stretching and Relaxation **131**

6.1	Upper back mobilization	132	6.2	Lateral back stretch	133
6.3	Pectoralis stretch	134	6.4	Latissimus stretch	135
6.5	Back mobilization	136	6.6	Pendulum	137
6.7	Sling splits	138			
6.8	Hip rotators (Internal rotation hips)				139
6.9	Hamstring stretch	140	6.10	Glute stretch	141
6.11	Quad stretch	142	6.12	Hip flexor stretch	143

7   Sport Specific Programs **145**

Credits 208

INTRODUCTION

Sling [sling] – Adjustable looped rope that increases demands on strength and balance compared to regular exercise. Ex: Sling Training, Sling Exercise.

I set my hands in the grips and get ready. Feet are shoulder width apart and my body in plank position. Sling push-ups – how hard can it be?

As I lower myself to the floor, I feel my hands starting to shake. I'm fighting to keep my balance. Chest, arms and core muscles are working at their maximum.

I concentrate to keep my hands steady. My pulse is racing, but I continue for another repetition. Do I always breathe this hard?

After seven reps I collapse on the floor. Seven push-ups? I'm supposed to do five times as many!

This was my first encounter with sling training. Now, what will sling training do for you?

Sling training is different. It will make you stronger. Faster. More flexible. It develops your balance. It can prevent sports injuries. You will feel improvements – whether you're running, golfing or rock climbing.

My only concern is that... you will get addicted.

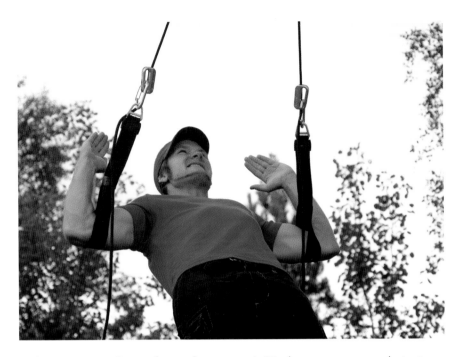

Welcome to an all new form of movement. We hope you are ready to try a workout that is suited to you – whatever your shape, height, weight or age. Sling training is a balanced, full body workout that delivers quicker results than regular machine training. It challenges strength, balance and joint stability at the same time. Most important of all, you will notice the results of sling training in your daily life.

Let's say you're moving to a new place and you'll be carrying boxes all day. When you lift a heavy box you need to be strong in all the body, not just the arms. The arms do only a part of the lifting; the shoulders, core and leg muscles do the rest.

Movement science has a term for this: muscle chains. Muscle chains are cooperating muscles that work together to perform different tasks like lifting, jumping, running or throwing. A chain is never stronger than its weakest link and the same applies to the muscle chains of the body.

A "balanced, full body workout" means that all the muscles are strengthened with the most stress on the weakest link. Strength machines and free weights will not strengthen your body the same way. The variable, wobbly support of the slings increase joint stability and decreases the risk of sport injuries. You will get stronger AND prevent injury!

Buy a sling trainer and you'll have a gym on the go with hundreds of exercises. No other equipment lets you customize your workout in the same way. You'll save time at the gym when you don't need to wait in line or walk between machines and then adjust the seat and weight stack. Get creative and make your own sling exercises by adding balance boards or extra weights. When you come up with a new exercise, let us know at www.slingexercise.com.

We've made this book to show you how fun and valuable sling training can be.

If you exercise at home, the sling trainer will give you full body strength training whenever you want it. Bring your sling trainer to the park or do a post-run sling routine in your garage.

If you are a gym member, sling training will give you the variation you need to get faster and better results. Challenge yourself and activate muscles you didn't know you have!

Why this book?

We started on this book to show you all the possibilities you have with a sling trainer. We want to give you:

▶ The best basic exercises
▶ Exercises for specific muscles and muscle groups
▶ Extreme sling training
▶ Stretching and flexibility exercises
▶ Workout routines and sport specific programs

Variation is the key to any workout. Even if you already have the perfect upper or lower body workout, we encourage you to add one or two sling exercises and notice the effect.

We rigorously test every sling exercise we find. This book is the premium selection of sling exercises. If you find an exercise that is missing, we'd love to hear from you at www.slingexercise.com.

Most sling exercises can be modified with equipment like a medicine ball, balance board, free weights or the Pilates ball. In a similar manner you may modify and exercise by shifting from toes to knees or changing from two to one hand for support.

With all the ways to modify an exercise there is an infinite number of variations. We will show you examples of these variations and hope you are inspired to make your own. Good news for personal trainers and instructors: We've made every exercise description independent of the photos. This way, the book will be valuable when helping out friends or instructing clients.

11

How did sling training start?

Several thousand years ago, gymnastics were started by the ancient Greeks. Physical fitness was encouraged and all Greek cities had a Gymnasium; a courtyard for exercise. The gymnastic rings, or still rings, were introduced by the Romans and used as part of military training. Some of the sling exercises are inspired by the moves done in gymnastic rings.

Slings have been used ever since for fun and for fitness gain. The earliest modern version of sling training is recorded in the book Athletic Sports For Boys published in 1866. This book provided several exercise suggestions and was the first book to describe sling training! By the end of the 1800s, there were several patents for various designs of sling trainers.

At the start of the 1900s, doctors and physical therapists started to use slings. Sling treatment or sling therapy is used to elevate a part of the body to provide friction-free movement. This "eliminates gravity" to let weak patients move their body parts freely for therapeutic movement and flexibility. In Chapter 6: Stretching, we use the same principle to let you relax and loosen stiff joints and muscle.

Sling therapy has been around for a long time, but sling training has resurfaced only in the past five years and has become increasingly popular. Sling training is spreading because of its reputation as a functional and valuable training tool.

Bodyweight resistance training enhances your bodily perception and gives noticeable results in daily life. There are a number of sling trainers available; we've chosen to use Jungle Sports "Liana" in this book.

Get started!

Myth: You need professional instruction to do sling training correctly.

Fact: Like all forms of exercise, you should know the basic principles to get the best results and avoid injury.

We recommend that you start by reading the section "Before You Start"

Sling exercises range from super easy to extremely hard. In this book we give you everything from the basics to the advanced so you can train at your level and be continuously challenged anew.

Start with the easy exercises. Learn the basics. All the advanced exercises build on the easy – so learn the easy ones with perfect form.

Good luck!

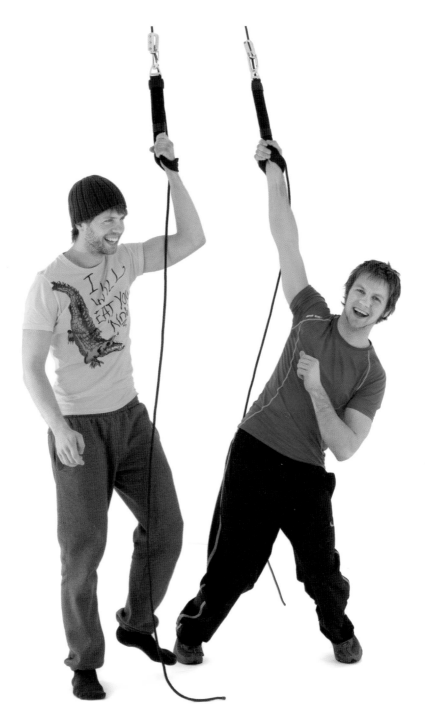

Authors Anders and Lennart in the studio.

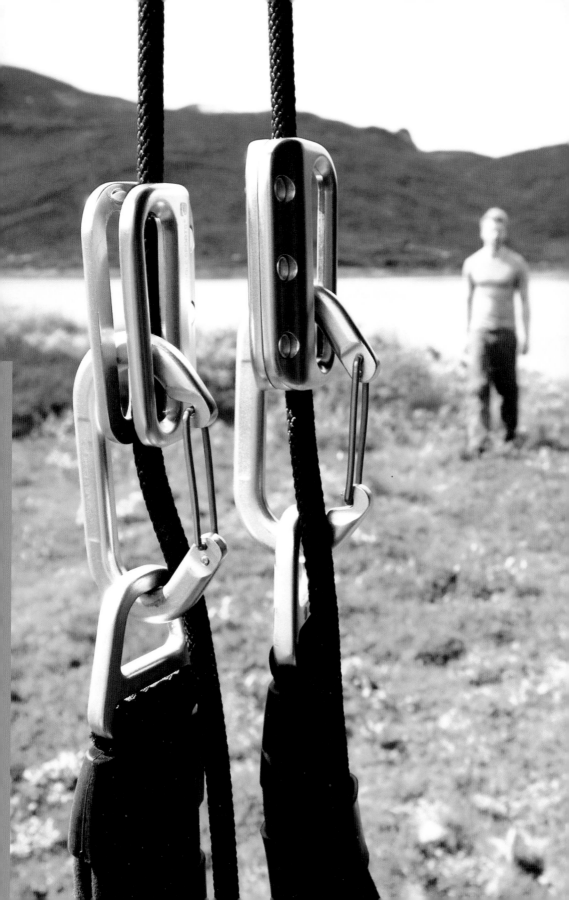

PART I

BEFORE YOU START

BEFORE YOU START

Sling training allows for a full body workout. From head to toes, you will work muscles you never knew you had.

Without any guidance, you may feel unsafe about good form, posture and heavy loads during sling training. And for maximum results, you want to train the right way. Through several years of instructing clients, we've boiled it down to three principles to master sling training:

- ▶ Perfect posture
- ▶ Core activation
- ▶ The 80/100 option

Perfect posture

If someone sees you doing a sling exercise, I want them to think: "Wow, this person is working out with perfect posture." Perfect posture is keeping your shoulders low, your neck relaxed, active abs and a neutral back posture. If you're training with perfect posture, there's a high chance you're doing it right!

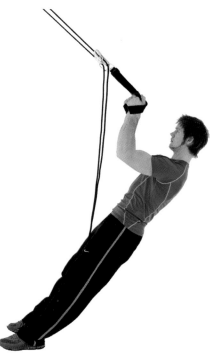

Core activation

In daily life we have two ways of cheating ourselves when standing or sitting. I am guilty of this myself: When standing, I get into a "duck pose," overarching my back and sticking out my butt. This allows me to relax my abs while the joints and ligaments of the back keep my upper body erect. It feels relaxing since I'm not contracting the abs, but after a while I'll feel the strain on the back and contract the abs.

The other way of cheating is in the sitting position. I will feel myself sliding forward in the chair and end up with a curved back, what is known as the "banana pose." This feels good because I am not using any back muscles, but resting on the ligaments and joints of the back. In the long run however, I'll get uncomfortable and sore in the back.

The abs should be active to avoid excessive overarching of the back. Whether sitting or standing, the back should be slightly curved in its neutral, correct posture.

The exercise on the next page is a simple way to find the neutral and correct posture. You will feel the lower part of your abs working to keep you in the neutral posture. When working out you should feel the abs contracting the same way as in this exercise.

The 80/100 option

In the exercise on the next page you'll notice that the last bit of stretching out the hips is the most demanding for the abs and back.

Keeping the hips straight can be exhausting and might discourage some people who think they can never be strong enough for sling training.

If you work out with hips slightly bent, you're exercising at 80 percent. It's easier on the core muscles and allows beginners to try more exercises without total fatigue.

There's nothing wrong with training at 80%. Starting out, hardly anyone can train at 100% in the slings, so begin at 80% and work your way up to 100%. When you are working with hips straight, you are at 100%. is a good way to feel the difference between working at 80 versus 100%.

If these three principles are too much, just remember this one rule:

When your abs are straining, you're doing it right. When your back is straining, you should take a break or choose an easier exercise.

Core stability

All sling training should be done with the correct posture and good form. This exercise will show you how to maintain a neutral spine and avoid strain.

Spinal movement

Lie on your back with your knees bent, as in the picture. Concentrate on your lower back and vary between increasing and straightening out the curve of the lower back. Your lower back should be curved just enough to slide your fingers

between your lower back and the floor. Engage the abdominal muscles so the lower back presses lightly on the fingers. This is the neutral position for the spine for correct posture.

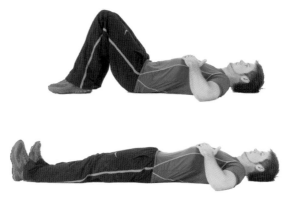

General tips

All sling training should be pain free. Stop the exercise immediately if you feel any discomfort or pain. Adjust the exercise to make it easier before you attempt to continue.

If you start to feel tiredness or strain in the low back, then either the exercise is too hard or your spine is not in the neutral position.

Keep shoulders low and relax the neck

Exercises will flow smoother and feel better if you keep your shoulders low and the neck in a neutral, relaxed position. The neck should be a natural extension of the spine.

The neutral position for the neck is the way the head rests on the neck when you are standing.

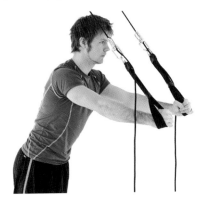

Hips over knees over toes

In lower body exercises, your hips, knees and toes should be in line. This applies to all leg exercises, not just sling training.

With the hips, knees and toes in line the joints receive equal pressure distribution and the muscle work is balanced. This will help prevent knee strain and injury.

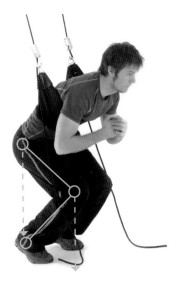

19

Plank core stability

CORRECT   Body is level from head to toe; spine is in the neutral position with a slight curve. Shoulders are at a 90 degree angle to the body.

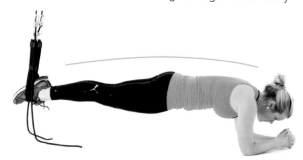

WRONG   Abs are not engaged, making the hips fall forward and causing excessive curving of the spine.

If you find yourself in this position, contract your abs, lift your hips and tilt the pelvis back.

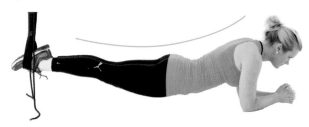

WRONG   The hips are piked up in the air.

This increases shoulder strain and promotes bad posture. Lower the hips and straighten the back to achieve the correct, neutral position.

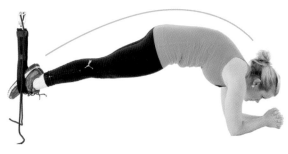

Standing core stability

CORRECT   Hips are straight and the back is in a neutral spine position. Arms are at 90 degrees to the body.

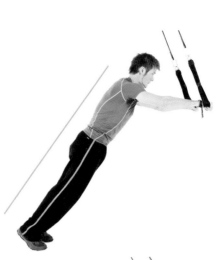

CORRECT   80%: The body is bent at the hips, butt sticking out. Straighten out the hips and return to a neutral spine position. Straighten out the hips to get a tougher challenge for the abs and back.

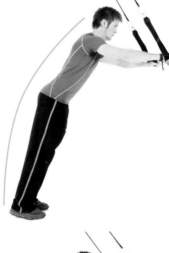

WRONG   Abs are not contracted, spine is curved and the hips fall forward. If you find yourself in this position, return to a neutral spine position.

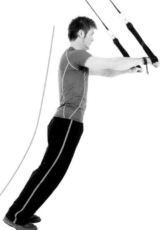

Sets and repetitions

What's the difference between numbers of repetitions, light and heavy load? How does it affect my results?

Repetitions (reps) – How many times you repeat a movement (exercise) before taking a break. If you are doing 8 repetitions, resistance should be adjusted so that you just manage these repetitions (not 9, 10 or more).

Sets – A group of repetitions of one exercise. After a set, you should take a one-minute break before you start again. Alternatively, you could do a superset.

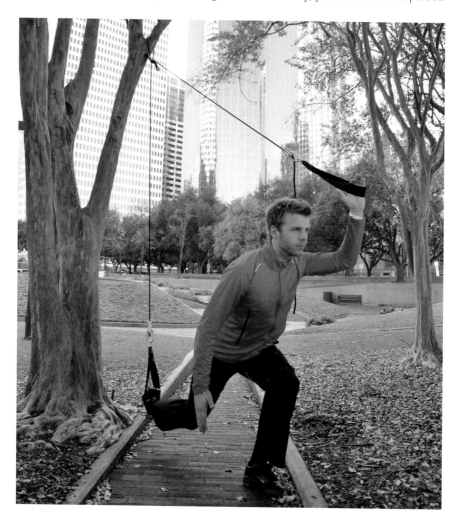

Superset (push-pull superset) – Alternating between two (or more) exercises without a break. This should be done with opposing muscle groups (e.g., chest/back) so one muscle group rests while the other is worked. This allows you to do your workout in half the time.

Dropset/Maxload/Pyramid set – A technique for continuing an exercise with a lower resistance once muscle failure has been achieved at a higher resistance. Example, when unable to complete another repetition with correct form for a low row exercise, take a step back, lower resistance and attempt another repetition. When you reach muscle failure, step back again (See also supporting foot, page 22).

Adjusting resistance

In regular weight training, resistance increases with increasing weights (e.g., heavier dumbbells or a larger weight stack). In sling training there are several options to increase resistance (see page 31).

Rep and set recommendations according to activity

Activity	Reps	Sets	Load
Warm up	Around 30	2	Light
Endurance strength	20-25	3	Medium
Muscle gain (hypertrophy)	10-12	4-8	Heavy
Max strength increase	4-6	3	Very Heavy

These are general recommendations. There are hundreds of rep-set schemes and magic lifting formulas all claiming to give better, faster results. Research has shown that simple rep-set schemes like the above are as efficient as any other*.

* Siff MC (2003). *Supertraining.* Supertraining Institute.

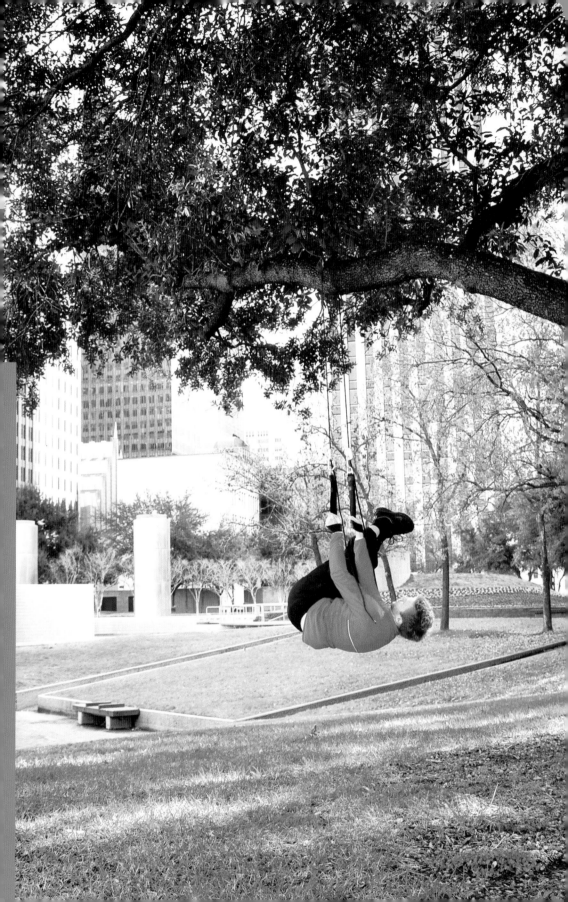

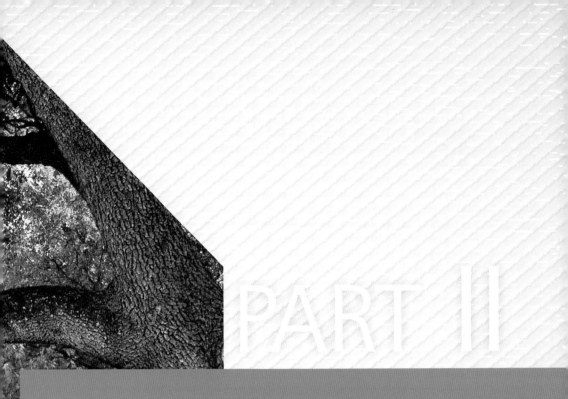

PART II

TO WORK OUT IN SLINGS

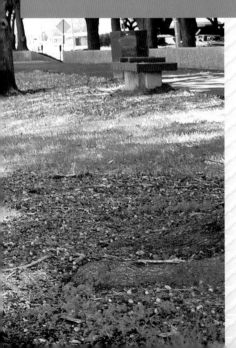

TO WORK OUT IN SLINGS

Basics: backward position

Adjust the sling trainer to the height indicated. An exercise gets harder the lower you adjust the slings.

You can adjust the demand put on the abs/back by bending or straightening your hip (see also the 80/100 option, page 17).

Stand two feet behind the sling attachment point. Exercises get harder as you step closer to where the slings are attached.

Lean back, supporting your body with extended arms. The arms should be 90 degrees to the body.

Keep the back in a neutral spine position.

Keep your body in a straight line. It's easy to "cheat" by pushing your hips forward when the exercises get tough.

Making an exercise easier or harder is as easy as taking a step backward or forward. Stepping forward makes a sharper angle between your body and the floor, increasing the amount of bodyweight you need to lift.

The closer your feet are to the point of sling attachment, the harder the exercise will be.

When you're at a sharp angle with the floor, your feet may start sliding forward. To prevent this, bend your knees so the entire sole of the foot makes contact with the floor.

When doing an exercise with knees bent, the back should still be in a neutral spine position. For an extra challenge you can try straightening the knees as you pull yourself up from the backward position.

27

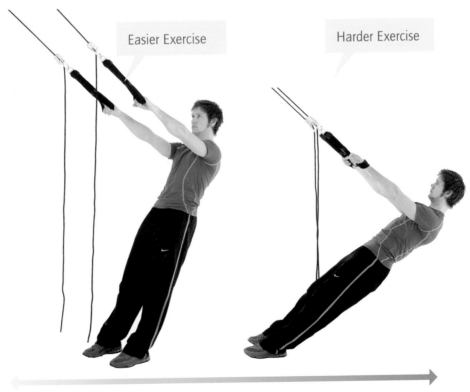

Easier Exercise

Harder Exercise

Easier

Harder

Forward position

Adjust the sling trainer to the height indicated. An exercise gets more challenging the lower you adjust the slings.

Lean forward, supporting your body on extended arms. The arms should be 90 degrees to the body.

Keep the back in a neutral spine position.

Keep your body in a straight line – it's easy to "cheat" by bending at the hips.

When exercising you should feel the abs working. If you start to feel strain, tiredness or pain in the lower back – stop immediately. Return to start. Make the exercise easier and find your neutral spine position.

Stand a foot or two in front of the point of sling attachment.

Making an exercise easier or harder is as easy as taking a step forward or backward. Stepping backward makes a sharper angle between your body and the floor, increasing the amount of bodyweight you have to lift.

The closer your feet are to the point of sling attachment, the harder your exercise will be.

As you get stronger and more experienced, you may be able to step back past the sling attachment!

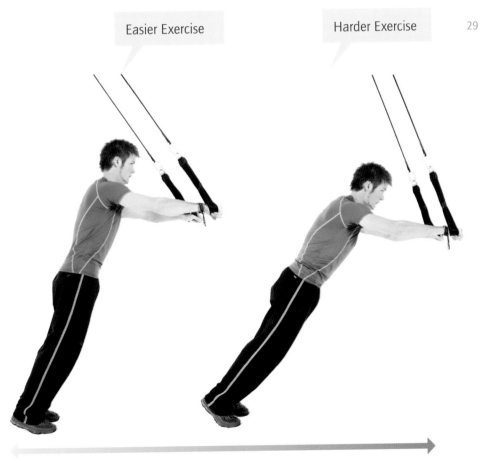

Easier Exercise

Harder Exercise

Easier

Harder

Supporting foot

Using one foot for extra support is beneficial if you are:

▶ Trying an exercise for the first time
▶ Feeling uncertain about an exercise
▶ Exercising by dropsets (see page 23)

To use a supporting foot, place one leg in front of the other while doing an exercise.

You may now use the supporting foot to push off and make an exercise easier. The supporting foot specifically reduces the demands on the core muscles. If you are doing an arm workout, using a supporting foot is a good technique to work your arms until muscle failure.

In the backward position

Place one foot behind the other, toes just touching the floor. Now the rear foot is available to push off during hard exercises. Maintain a neutral spine position and a straight body through the hips.

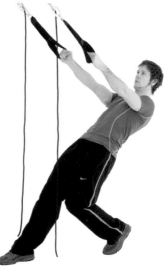

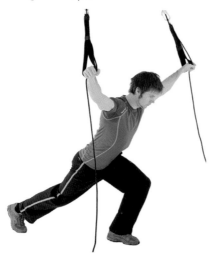

In the forward position

Place one foot in front of the other. If an exercise is too hard, use the front foot to push off of the floor. Maintain a neutral spine position and the body in a straight line.

One of the great advantages of sling training is adjusting the resistance to fit your level. Here are some ways to increase difficulty that may be applied to any exercise.

1. Move backward
2. Lower sling height
3. Exercise on one leg
4. Use an unstable surface

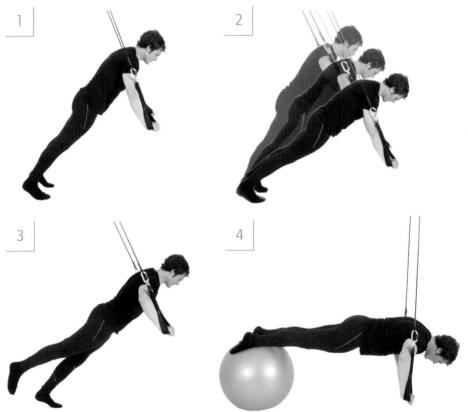

There are several other ways to make an exercise easier or harder, depending on the equipment available. An incline board, weight belt or pulleys can make exercises even more challenging.

Sling training is developing fast with new exercises and combinations of sling trainers and other equipment appearing all the time. To see the latest developments and exercises, check out our blog at www.slingexercise.com.

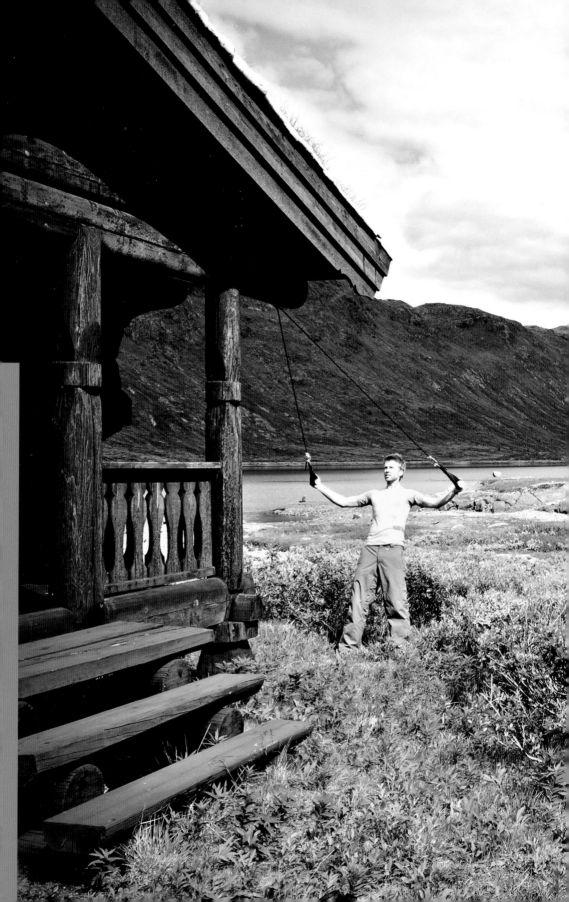

PART III

GET THE MOST
OUT OF THE BOOK

III

GET THE MOST OUT OF THE BOOK

Know your way around

In the description you'll find a thorough explanation on how to do the exercises. Below the text you'll find illustrative pictures. When learning a new exercise, you should first try the start and end position independently before moving through the exercise.

Start position

Before you begin, notice your position relative to the sling attachment. Will this be an easy exercise or a hard one? You choose where you place yourself. Make sure your back is in the neutral spine position.

End position

The rightmost picture on a page always illustrates the end position of the exercise. Check the muscle diagram to see if you are working the targeted muscles when you are in this position.

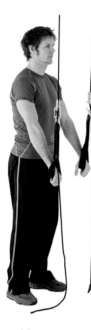
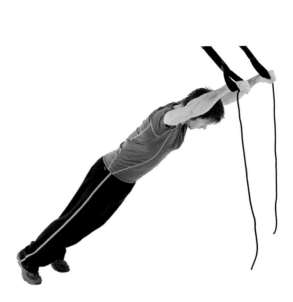

start position   *end position*

3.24 Pull-ups

Reach and grasp the slings with a wide overhand grip. Lift your feet off the ground. Crossing is optional. Using your arms, lift your body until the chin is the same height as your hands. Lower body until arms are straight.

Expert advice: Avoid locking the elbows when the arms are straight by keeping ready tension in the biceps and shoulders.

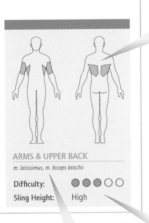

ARMS & UPPER BACK
m. latissimus, m. biceps brachii

Difficulty: ●●●○○
Sling Height: High

Feel and see the muscles working

On every exercise page you'll find the primary muscles marked in green. Because all sling training engages the core muscles, only the main muscles for a given exercise are marked green in the diagram. When exercising, you should feel these muscles working.

Expert advice

This section features tips on how to improve form and avoid common mistakes. Also, look for new ways for variation in this section

Musculus pectoralis

Main muscles are named in Latin for international reference. This is also handy for personal trainers and anatomy buffs.

Difficulty-Level & Sling-Height

see next pages

Sling height

Beneath the name of the exercise you will find a suggested sling height.

You will want more challenge as you progress through exercises. Lowering the sling height will make any exercise more difficult.

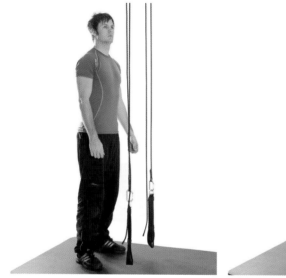

Ankle

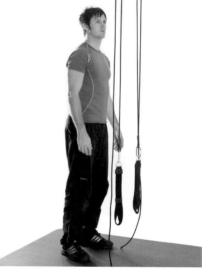

Leg

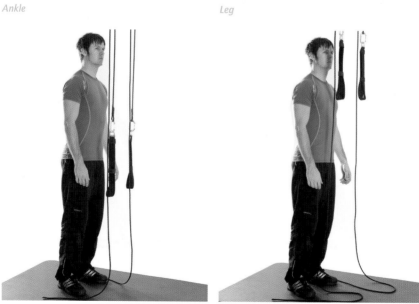

Thigh

Chest

Difficulty level

Side by side with the sling height, you'll find the difficulty level. This is a subjective measure from 1 to 5, based on both the technical challenge and muscular strength needed for the exercise.

Low level of difficulty

The exercise is easy to learn and does not require great strength, coordination or balance. Any sling exercise can be made hard – but at the current settings this exercise has a low level of difficulty.

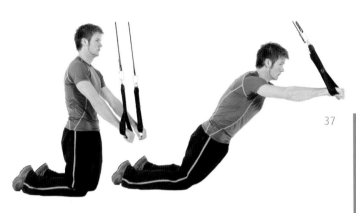

37

High level of difficulty

The exercise places great demands on muscular strength, coordination or balance. The exercise cannot be made easier and should only be attempted by experienced students of sling training.

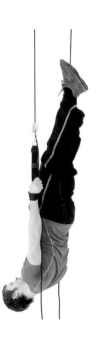

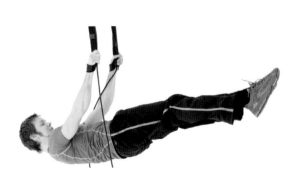

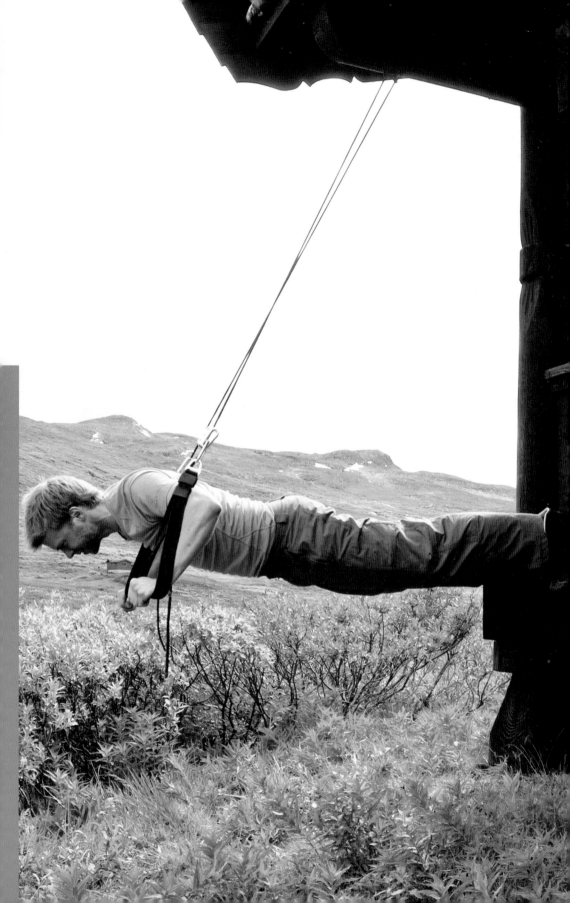

EXERCISES
FULL BODY WORKOUT

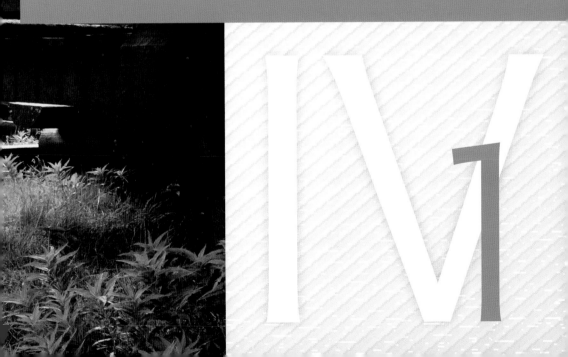

Chapter 1

FULL BODY WORKOUT

1.1   Squat and row

Start in the backward position. Lean back on extended arms and bend your knees to a deep squat. Hold this position for a second. Now pull the slings toward you, catapulting up from the squat and driving the elbows back and out to the sides. Repeat.

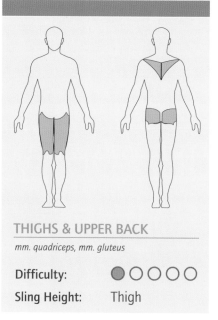

THIGHS & UPPER BACK
mm. quadriceps, mm. gluteus

Difficulty: ●○○○○
Sling Height: Thigh

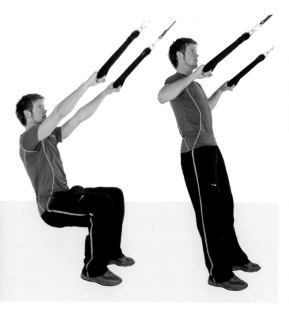

Expert advice: Try varying the way you pull yourself up from the deep squat. The harder you pull on the slings, the more you'll be working the upper back. Pointing the elbows out to the sides will work the shoulder blade muscles specifically.

1.2   Lunge and fly

Start in the forward position. Take a big step forward. Squat down until the forward knee is at 90 degrees, and stretch out the arms with elbows to the side. Push off with forward leg and bring arms together in a hugging motion to return to starting position. Repeat with opposite leg in front.

Expert advice: You should feel a stretch in the chest muscles when in the end position. For variation, try stretching your arms out overhead instead of stretching out to the side.

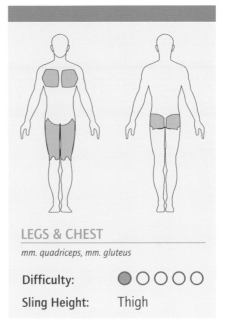

LEGS & CHEST
mm. quadriceps, mm. gluteus

Difficulty: ●○○○○
Sling Height: Thigh

41

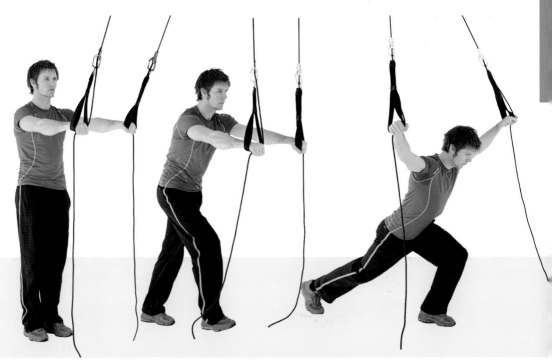

1.3   Lunge with side bend

Start in a forward position. Take a big step forward. Squat down until the forward knee is at 90 degrees and bend the upper body to the same side as the knee. You should feel a stretch in the opposite side of the upper body. Push off with your forward leg, straighten out the back and return to starting position. Repeat with opposite leg, bending the upper body to the opposite side.

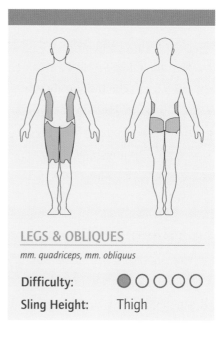

LEGS & OBLIQUES
mm. quadriceps, mm. obliquus

Difficulty: ●○○○○

Sling Height: Thigh

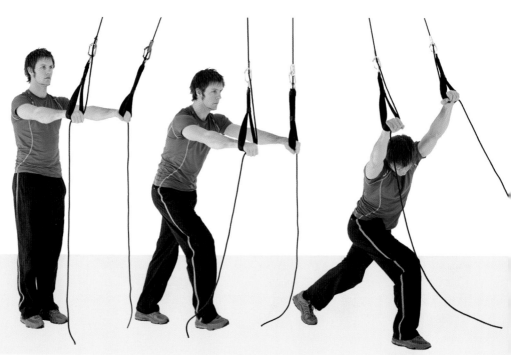

1.4 One leg squat to lunge

Start in the backward position. Lift one leg off the floor and bend the knee of the other into a one leg squat (see exercise 2.1). From this position, pull yourself up and forward into a lunge (setting the floating foot down in front). Use your arms and the forward leg to push back to start. Repeat with opposite leg.

Expert advice: Start far behind the position of sling attachment to avoid ending up too far in front of the sling attachment at the end of the exercise.

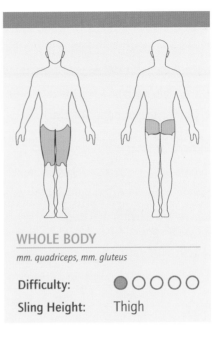

WHOLE BODY

mm. quadriceps, mm. gluteus

Difficulty:	●○○○○
Sling Height:	Thigh

43

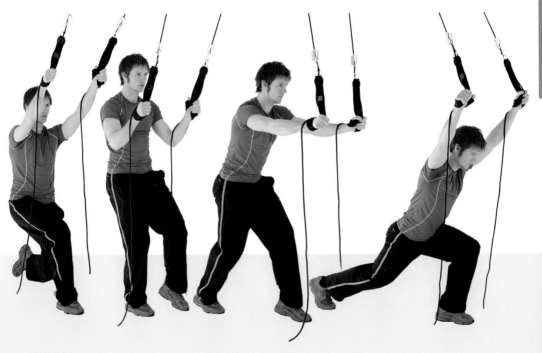

1.5　Overhead boxing

Begin in a forward position. Bend your knees and reach the right arm up and over to the left side. As your right hand shoots up, extend the knees to standing. Repeat for opposite arm.

Expert advice: This exercise is done dynamically – no rest between repetitions. Imagine boxing towards the roof as you are moving nonstop.

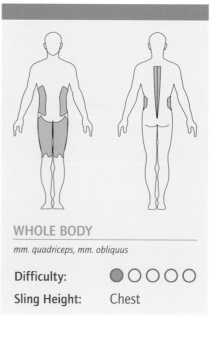

WHOLE BODY

mm. quadriceps, mm. obliquus

Difficulty: ●○○○○

Sling Height:　Chest

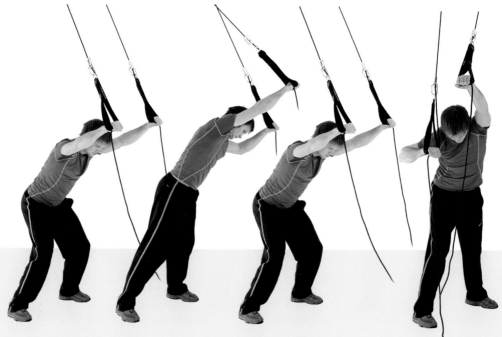

1.6 Ice skates

Start in the backward position. Use hands in slings for support while crossing your legs from side to side. Let the back leg cross behind the standing leg, then drive the standing leg far out to the side. Bend the knee and kick back to the starting position like an ice skater. Repeat to the opposite side.

Expert advice: Work dynamically; make this a flowing movement from side to side.

GLUTES & THIGHS

mm. quadriceps, mm. gluteus

Difficulty: ●○○○○

Sling Height: Thigh

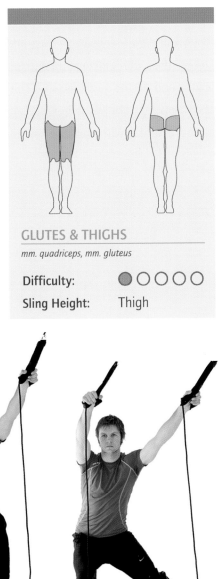

1.7   Sprinter start

Lie forward supported in a wide sling, feet on the ground. Load one leg and kick off the ground moving up and forward. Land on the same leg in a controlled manner and return to starting position. Repeat with opposite leg.

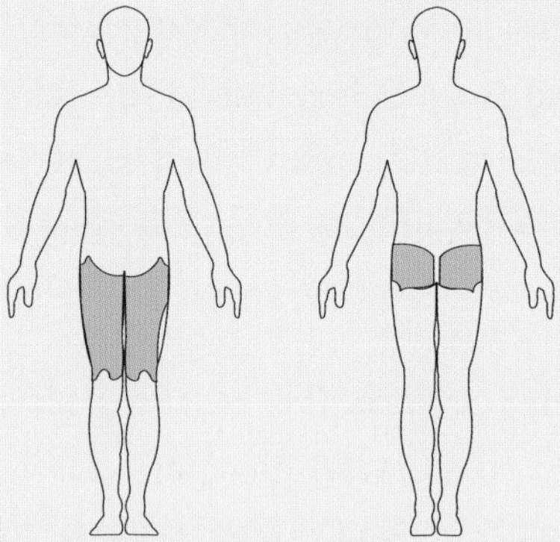

GLUTES & THIGHS

mm. quadriceps, mm. gluteus

Difficulty: ●○○○○

Sling Height: Thigh

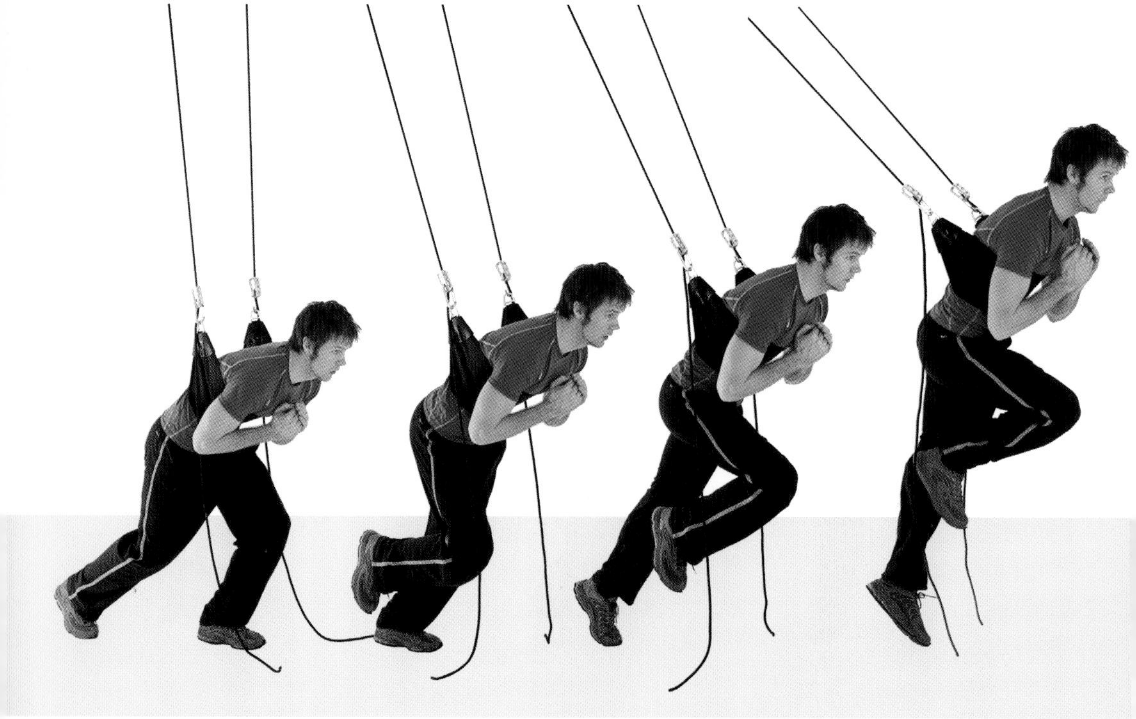

1.8　Postural squat

Start in the backward position. Lift arms straight overhead with palms facing forward. Maintain tension in the slings as you squat down to 90 degrees. Hold for a second before returning to start.

Expert advice: This exercise promotes good posture and strengthens the legs, upper back and shoulders. The perfect exercise for office workers!

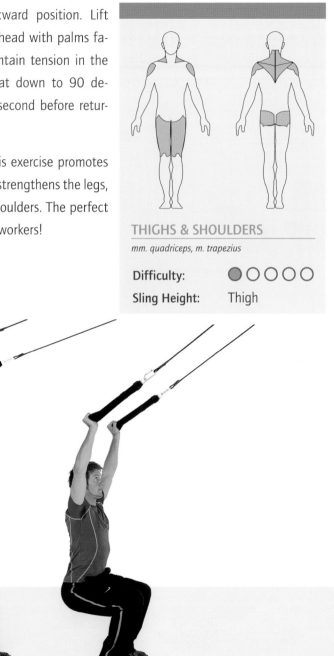

THIGHS & SHOULDERS

mm. quadriceps, m. trapezius

Difficulty:　⬤〇〇〇〇

Sling Height:　Thigh

47

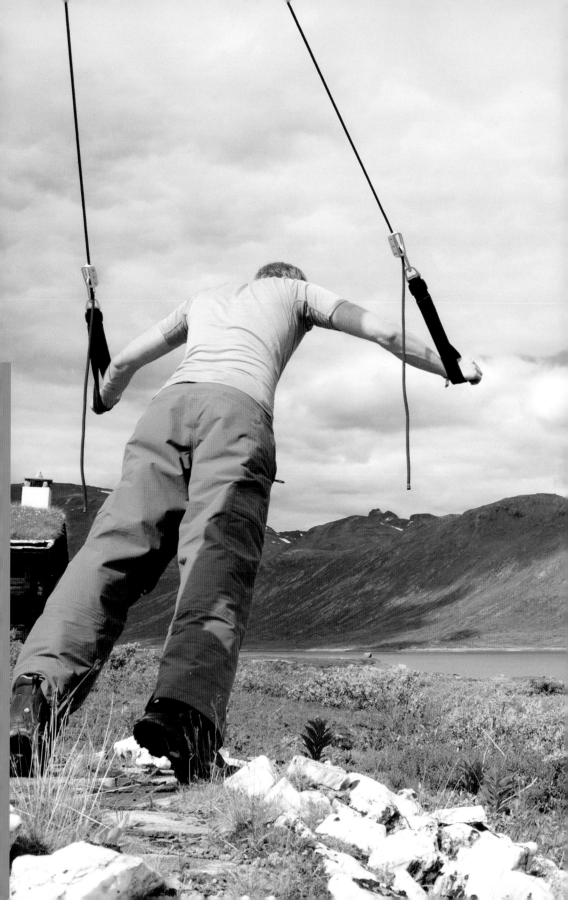

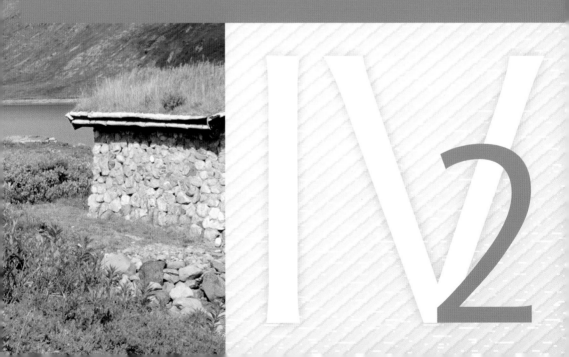

PART IV

CHAPTER 2

EXERCISES
LOWER BODY STRENGTH

IV

IV 2

Chapter 2

LOWER BODY STRENGTH

2.1 One leg squat

Stand in the backward position. Lift one leg off the floor; bend the other until the knee is at 90 degrees. Straighten out the knee and return to starting position. You should use your hands in the slings only to keep balance in this exercise.

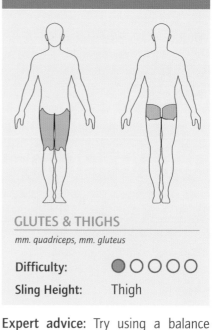

GLUTES & THIGHS
mm. quadriceps, mm. gluteus

Difficulty: ●○○○○
Sling Height: Thigh

Expert advice: Try using a balance board as a support surface to work your knee-ankle stability.

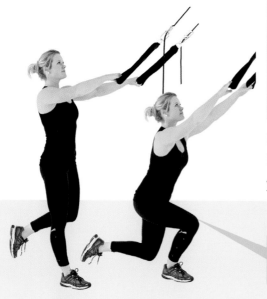

Remember to keep the hip, knee and toes in a straight line (see page 19)

2.2   One leg squat with rotation

Perform the exercise as described on the previous page (2.1), but turn your back leg inward (rotate the back leg in toward the opposite leg).

Expert advice: This rotation works the glutes specifically, making this one of the best butt lifting exercises. For progress, try using a balance board as a support surface.

The leg rotates back and in under the standing foot.

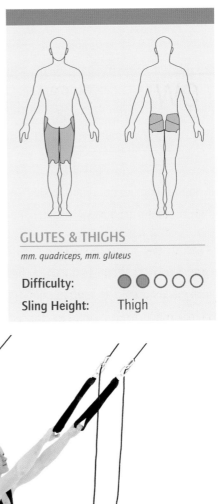

GLUTES & THIGHS

mm. quadriceps, mm. gluteus

Difficulty: ● ● ○ ○ ○

Sling Height: Thigh

51

Remember to keep the hip, knee and toes in a straight line (see page 19)

2.3 Backward lunge

Stand right underneath the sling attachment. One sling should be at ankle height, the other at chest height. Put one foot in the lower sling. Grab a hold of the other sling for support. Jump two steps forward and you're ready to start.

Push the sling leg backward while bending the front knee to 90 degrees. Return in a controlled manner.

Expert advice: When you master this exercise, let go of the support sling for a challenge to your balance.

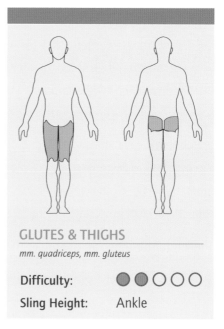

GLUTES & THIGHS
mm. quadriceps, mm. gluteus

Difficulty: ●●○○○
Sling Height: Ankle

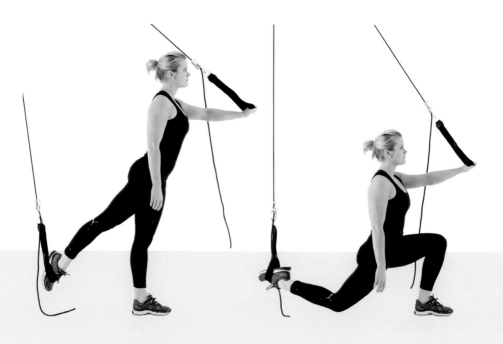

2.4　Backward lunge to jump

Start with a backward lunge (exercise 2.3). Following through the lunge, kick off the ground into a jump. Make a cushioned landing by bending the knee and go straight into a new backward lunge.

Expert advice: Want to work the glutes even more? While doing the backward lunge, try fully extending the back leg for each repetition.

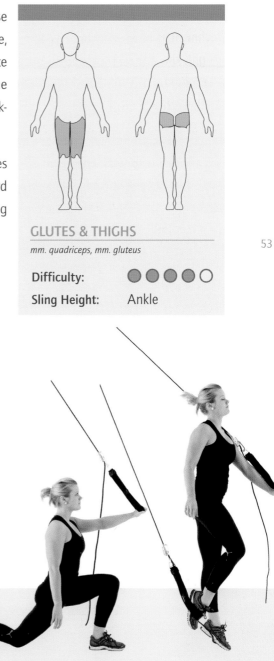

GLUTES & THIGHS

mm. quadriceps, mm. gluteus

Difficulty:	●●●●○
Sling Height:	Ankle

53

2.5   Stability lunge

Set one foot in the wide sling. Lean forward and bend your back knee to 90 degrees. Concentrate and balance in the end position for five seconds before returning to start.

Expert advice: The main purpose of this exercise is to work knee joint stability. The movement is best done in a wide sling – in a regular sling the rope may get in the way of your knee.

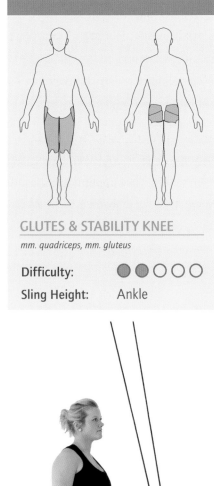

GLUTES & STABILITY KNEE

mm. quadriceps, mm. gluteus

Difficulty: ●●○○○

Sling Height: Ankle

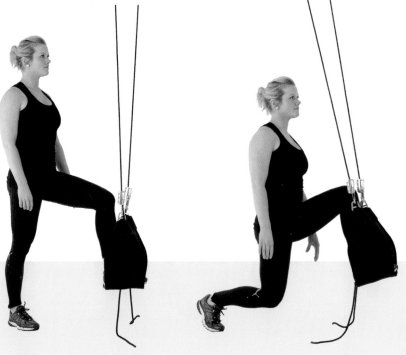

2.6   One leg deep squat

Start in the backward position. Lift and extend one leg in front of you while bending the knee of the other. Go as deep as your knee will allow before returning to standing.

Expert advice: Deep squats should only be done if you have strong leg muscles and are without any knee problems. If you are unsure, try the regular one leg squat (exercise 2.1) and work your way down gradually to the deep squat.

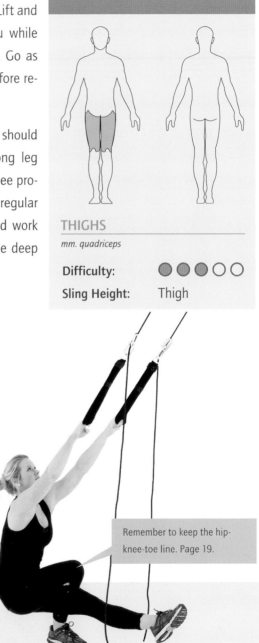

THIGHS
mm. quadriceps

Difficulty: ●●●○○

Sling Height: Thigh

55

Remember to keep the hip-knee-toe line. Page 19.

2.7 Hamstring curl

Lie on your back with heels in slings. Keep your back in the neutral spine position and lift your backside off the floor. Draw your feet toward you while keeping the back and hips in place.

Expert advice: To keep your calf muscles from cramping, angle your toes toward you as if you were walking on your heels.

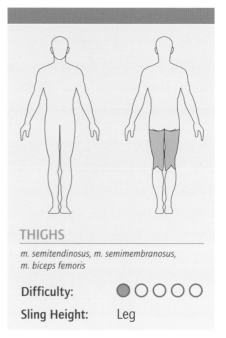

THIGHS

m. semitendinosus, m. semimembranosus, m. biceps femoris

Difficulty: ●○○○○

Sling Height: Leg

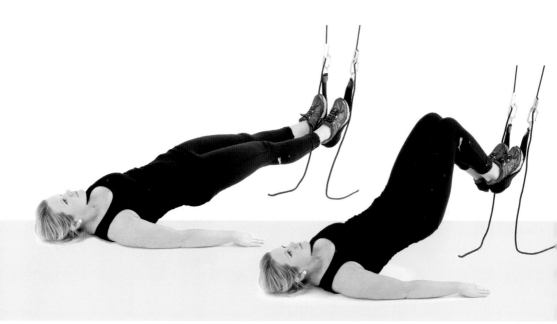

2.8   High hamstring curl

Perform the exercise like regular hamstring curls (exercise 2.7), but lift your hips as you draw your feet toward you. This variation is more challenging for the muscles of the back and thighs.

Expert advice: To keep your calf muscles from cramping, angle your toes toward you as if you were walking on your heels.

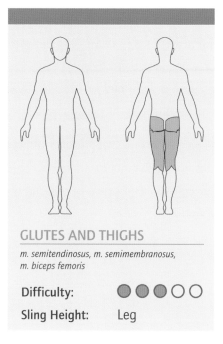

GLUTES AND THIGHS

*m. semitendinosus, m. semimembranosus,
m. biceps femoris*

Difficulty: ●●●○○

Sling Height: Leg

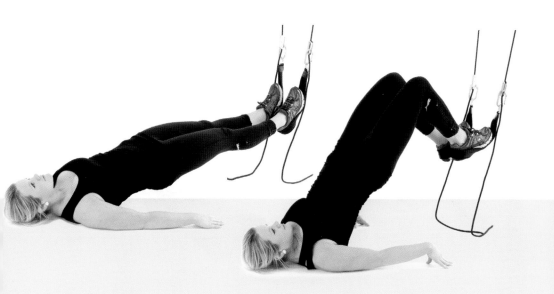

2.9   One leg hamstring curl

Perform the exercise like regular hamstring curls (exercise 2.7), but with only one leg supported in a sling. Engage your core muscles to keep from dipping down on the unsupported side.

Expert advice: To keep your calf muscles from cramping up, angle your toes towards you as if you were walking on your heels.

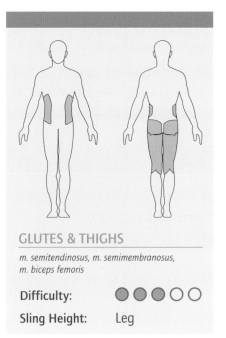

GLUTES & THIGHS

m. semitendinosus, m. semimembranosus, m. biceps femoris

Difficulty: ●●●○○

Sling Height: Leg

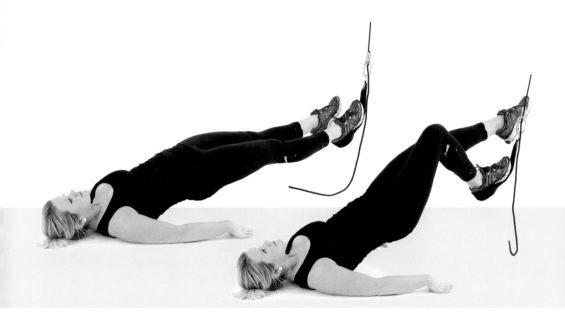

2.10 High extension to splits

Lie on your back with heels in slings. Keep your back in the neutral spine position and lift the hips off the floor. Spread your legs and hold for one second. You should feel the outside of your thighs working. Return to starting position, keeping your backside off the floor.

Expert advice: DO NOT do this exercise if you have any pelvic problems.

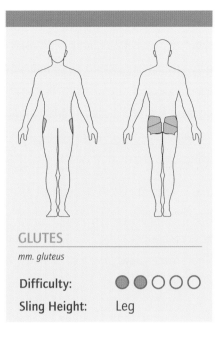

GLUTES

mm. gluteus

Difficulty:	●●○○○
Sling Height:	Leg

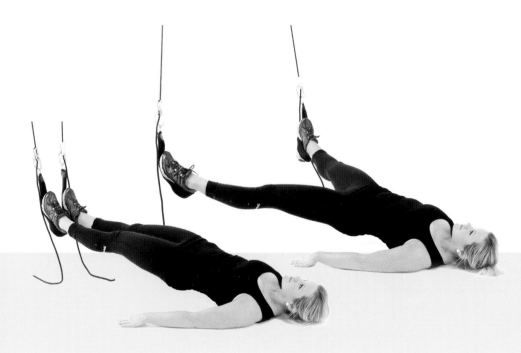

2.11   Sling leg lifts

Lie sideways with both feet in the wide sling. Lift your hips going into a sideways plank. Shoulders, hips and legs should be on a straight line. From this position, lift the upper leg and hold for three second before lowering. Keep your toes pointing forward; rotating your leg upwards is cheating!

Expert advice: Start easy with the wide sling above the knees. Move the sling farther down the leg to increase difficulty.

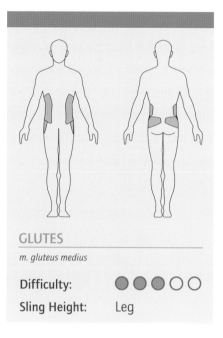

GLUTES

m. gluteus medius

Difficulty: ●●●○○

Sling Height: Leg

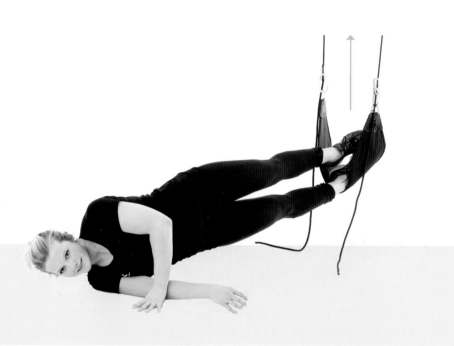

2.12   Inner thigh lifts

Lie sideways with your upper leg in the wide sling. Lift the hips and lower leg to form a sideways plank. Shoulders, hips and legs should be in a straight line. Hold for three seconds before lowering to the floor. Keep your toes pointing forward; rotating your leg upward is cheating!

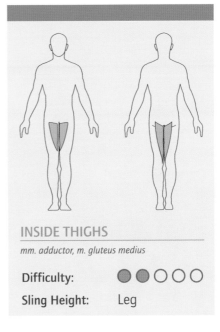

INSIDE THIGHS

mm. adductor, m. gluteus medius

Difficulty:　●●○○○

Sling Height:　　Leg

61

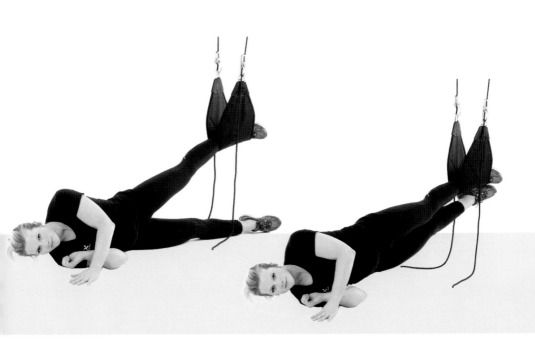

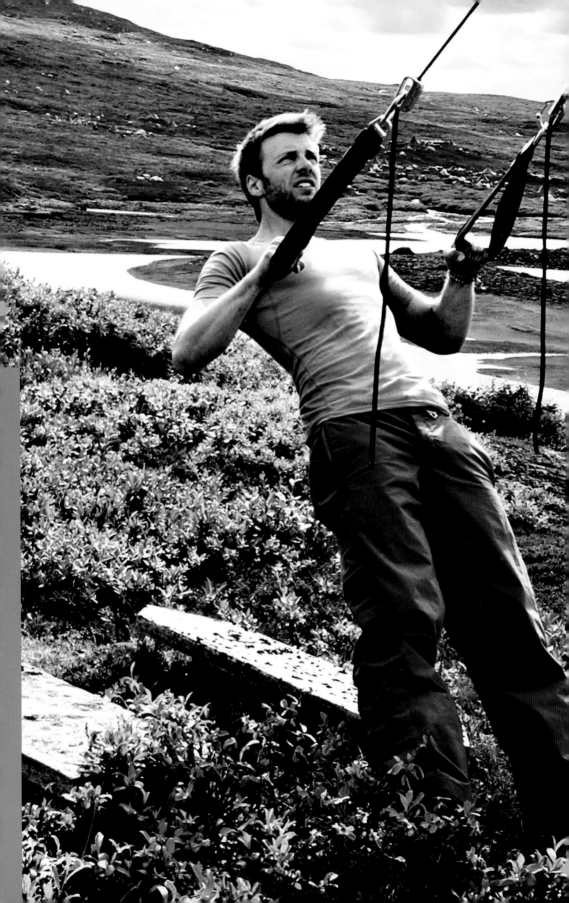

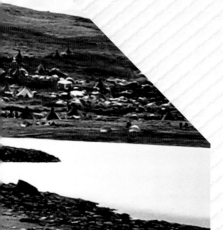

EXERCISES
UPPER BODY STRENGTH

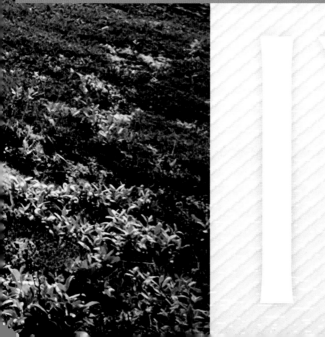
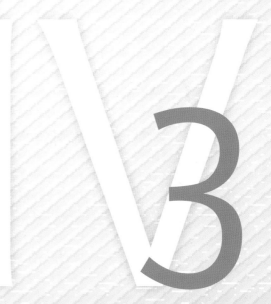

IV

3

Chapter 3

UPPER BODY STRENGTH

3.1   Kneeling superman

Grab on to the slings while kneeling. Your palms should be facing the floor. Lean forward and stretch your hands out in front of you. Hold for three seconds before pushing back to the starting position.

Expert advice: Concentrate on keeping your back in the neutral spine position and your shoulders down low and relaxed.

STABILITY SHOULDER & BACK

m. latissimus, m. rectus abdominis

| Difficulty: | ●○○○○ |
| Sling Height: | Leg |

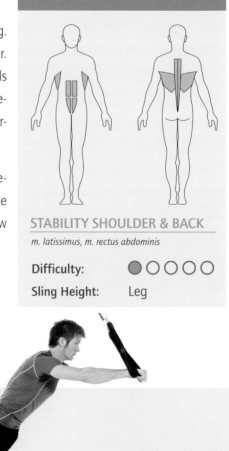

3.2   Superman

Grab on to the slings with your palms facing the floor. Lean forward supported by the arms. Keep leaning forward and stretch your hands over your head. Hold for three seconds before pushing back to the starting position.

Expert advice: Concentrate on keeping your back in the neutral spine position and your shoulders down low and relaxed. For an easier exercise, move the slings up past the elbows.

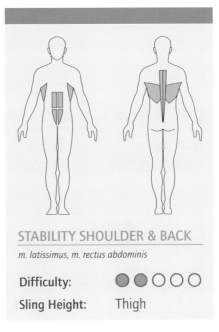

STABILITY SHOULDER & BACK
m. latissimus, m. rectus abdominis

Difficulty: ●●○○○

Sling Height: Thigh

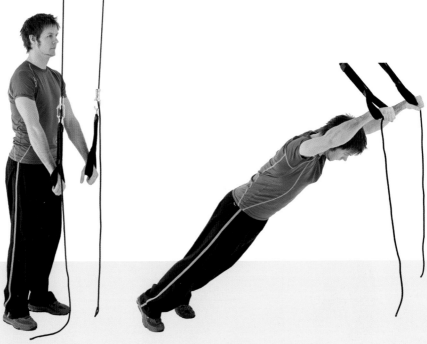

3.3 One hand superman

Like regular superman (exercise 3.2) but with only one hand for support. To avoid rotating your upper body, place yourself one step to the side of the sling you are holding on to.

Expert advice: This is a good exercise for the external obliques – the muscles shaping your waistline.

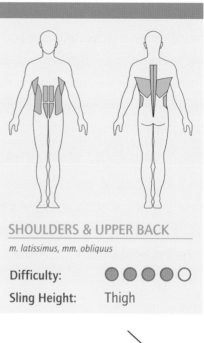

SHOULDERS & UPPER BACK

m. latissimus, mm. obliquus

Difficulty:	●●●●○
Sling Height:	Thigh

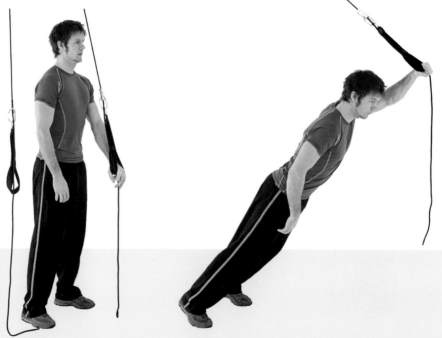

3.4 Flies

Start in the forward position. Keep elbows slightly bent and pointing backward. Lean forward and let the arms move out to the side. You should feel a stretch across the chest muscles. Hold for a second, then push off and bring your hands together in a hugging motion.

Expert advice: Keep the back in a neutral spine position. Engage the abs and keep your back straight.

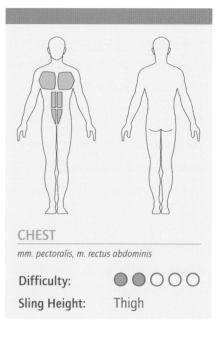

CHEST

mm. pectoralis, m. rectus abdominis

Difficulty: ●●○○○

Sling Height: Thigh

67

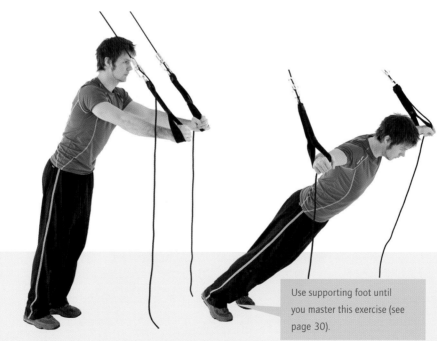

Use supporting foot until you master this exercise (see page 30).

3.5   Reverse elbow flies

Start in the backward position with the slings attached above the elbows. Keep the elbows bent at 90 degrees and straight in front of you.

Drive the body forward by pressing the arms out to the sides. Return slowly to the starting position. Keep the arms up high throughout – this is not the Low Row exercise.

Expert advice: For a harder exercise you may cross the slings. Place the left sling around the right elbow and the right sling around the left elbow to increase resistance.

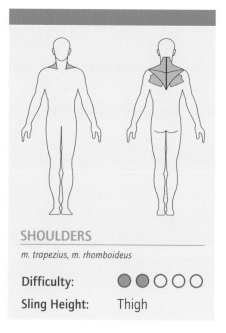

SHOULDERS

m. trapezius, m. rhomboideus

Difficulty: ●●○○○
Sling Height: Thigh

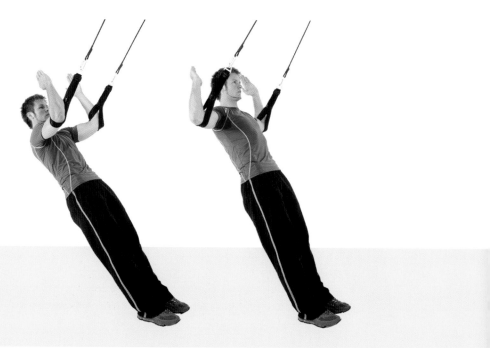

3.6   Reverse flies

Start in the backward position. Keep elbows slightly bent and elbow tips pointing backward. Drive the body forward by pressing the arms out to the side. Arms should be pointing in opposite directions at end position. Return slowly to starting position.

Expert advice: For a harder exercise you may cross the slings. Place the left sling in your right hand, right sling in your left hand. Remember to keep your back in the neutral spine position throughout.

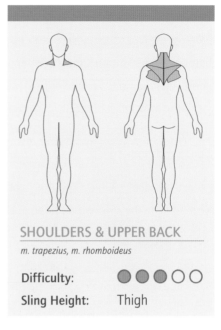

SHOULDERS & UPPER BACK

m. trapezius, m. rhomboideus

Difficulty: ●●●○○

Sling Height: Thigh

69

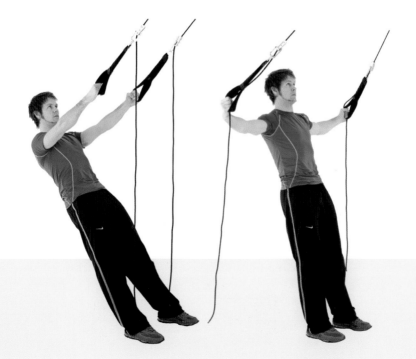

3.7   Y-flies

Start in the backward position, slings fastened around the wrists, not holding on. Keep elbows slightly bent and elbow tips pointing backward. Press your arms upward, ending in a Y-position, arms overhead. Return slowly to starting position.

Expert advice: Avoid cheating by pushing your hips forward. Keep the back in a neutral spine position.

SHOULDERS & UPPER ARMS

m. trapezius, m. deltoideus

Difficulty: ●●●○○

Sling Height: Thigh

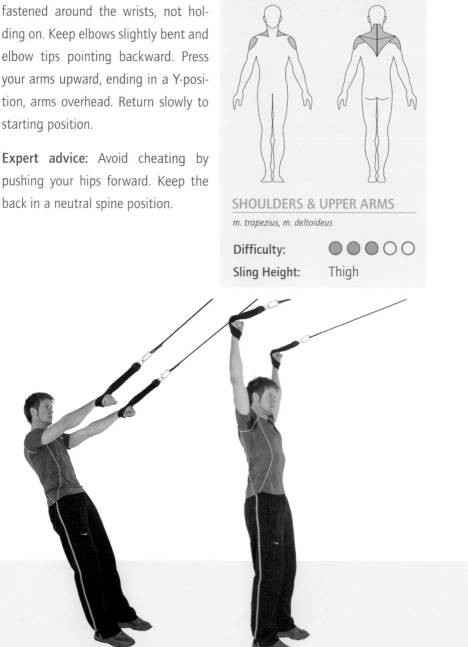

3.8   A-flies

Start in the backward position. Keep elbows slightly bent and the elbows pointing to the sides. Drive the body forward by pressing the arms downward. Lead with the chest and upper body concentrating, on keeping a neutral spine position. Release and bring the body back to the starting position.

SHOULDERS & UPPER BACK

m. trapezius, m. latissimus

Difficulty: ●●●○○

Sling Height: Thigh

71

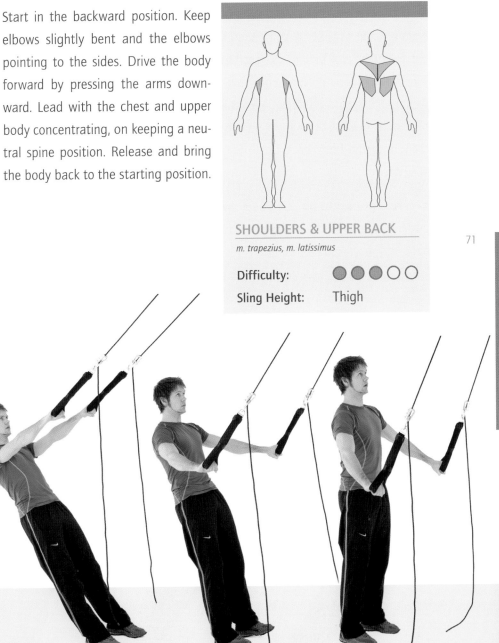

3.9 One arm row

Begin in the backward position, with one arm holding on to a sling. Stretch out the other arm behind you so that your arms are pointing in opposite directions. Pull yourself up and reach the back arm forward. Hold for a second, then lower the body back to starting position.

Expert advice: Avoid cheating by pushing your hips forward. Keep the back in a neutral spine position.

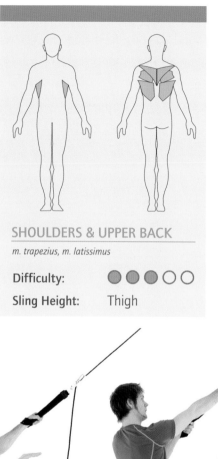

SHOULDERS & UPPER BACK

m. trapezius, m. latissimus

Difficulty: ●●●○○

Sling Height: Thigh

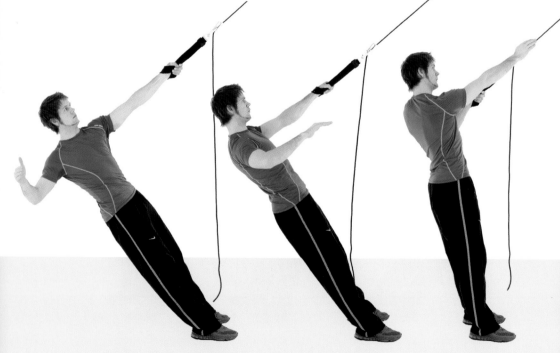

3.10 Incline pull-ups

Begin in the backward position. Keep shoulders low, chest pushed forward. Lift yourself up by pulling the elbows down and out to the sides. Release back down and repeat.

Expert advice: This exercise works the upper back specifically. For a lower back workout, pull up with the elbows close to the body. Place your feet on a balance board or fitness ball to make the exercise harder.

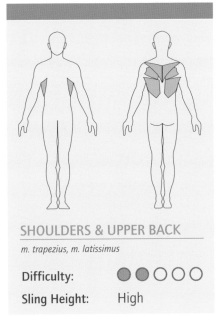

SHOULDERS & UPPER BACK
m. trapezius, m. latissimus

Difficulty: ●●○○○

Sling Height: High

73

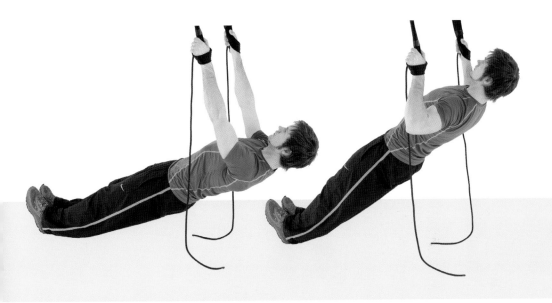

3.11   Bent arm side press

Stand sideways with one sling in your hand, elbow raised to 90 degrees and shoulder rotated inward. Lean toward the sling, drawing the elbow up over shoulder height. Hold for a second, then return to starting position.

Expert advice: This is a heavy isometric internal rotation exercise.

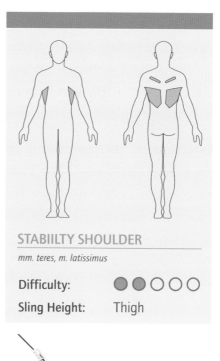

STABIILTY SHOULDER

mm. teres, m. latissimus

Difficulty: ●●○○○

Sling Height: Thigh

Bend the knee as you are leaning into the sling. Adjust the difficulty of the exercise by the amount you push off with your foot (See supporting foot, page 30).

3.12 Side press

Stand sideways with one sling in your hand. Lean into the sling on a straight arm, engaging the shoulder to keep your balance. Push downward to return to the starting position.

Expert advice: Keep your shoulder low throughout the movement. This is an excellent stability exercise for the shoulder.

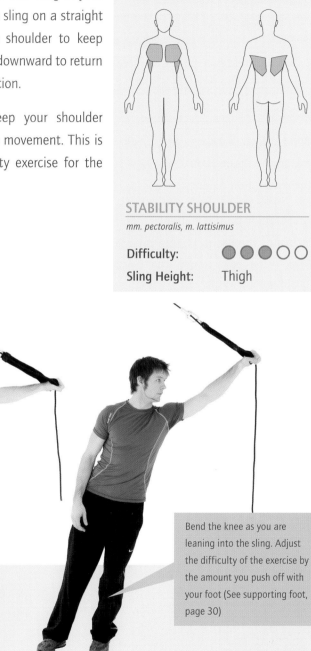

STABILITY SHOULDER

mm. pectoralis, m. lattisimus

Difficulty: ●●●○○

Sling Height: Thigh

75

Bend the knee as you are leaning into the sling. Adjust the difficulty of the exercise by the amount you push off with your foot (See supporting foot, page 30)

3.13 External rotation

Start in the backward position, holding on to the slings. Lift elbows to shoulder height and point them out to opposite directions. This is the starting position.

Keeping the elbows in a fixed position, rotate arms to bring your body forward. Hold for a second, then release back down bringing your body back to starting position.

Expert advice: To additionally work the extensor muscles of the forearm, fasten the slings around the wrists instead of holding on.

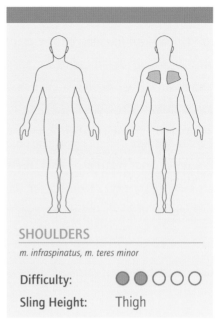

SHOULDERS

m. infraspinatus, m. teres minor

Difficulty: ●●○○○

Sling Height: Thigh

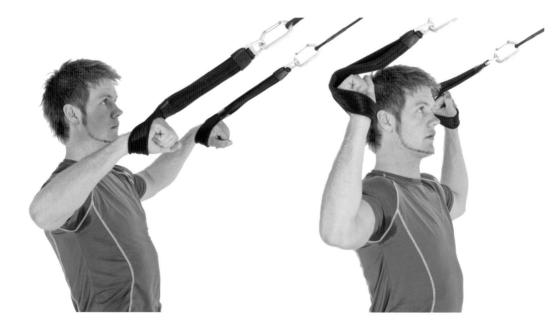

3.14 Internal rotation

Start in the forward position. Keep your shoulders low, the elbows high and pointing out to opposite sides. Lean forward by rotating arms upward, keeping your elbows in a fixed position. Hold for a second, then rotate by pressing arms downward and return to starting position.

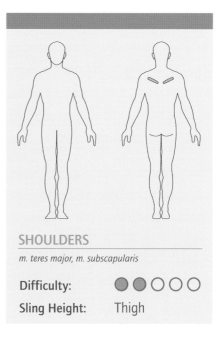

SHOULDERS

m. teres major, m. subscapularis

Difficulty: ●●○○○

Sling Height: Thigh

77

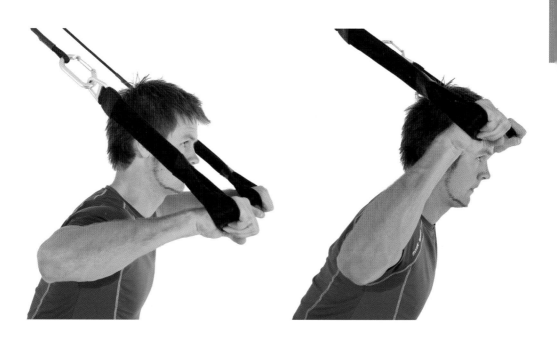

3.15 Hammer curls

Start in the backward position. Turn the arms so your thumbs face up. Keep your upper arms fixed in this position, and pull yourself forward by bending at the elbows. Hold for a second and sink back to starting position.

Expert advice: Keeping the upper arms fixed requires actively pushing the arms upward while you are performing the exercise. To get a feel for the correct position for the arms, try the correct start and end positions before attempting the exercise.

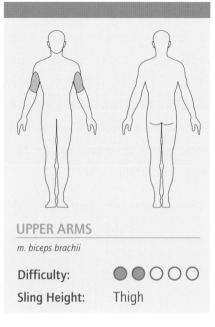

UPPER ARMS

m. biceps brachii

Difficulty: ●●○○○

Sling Height: Thigh

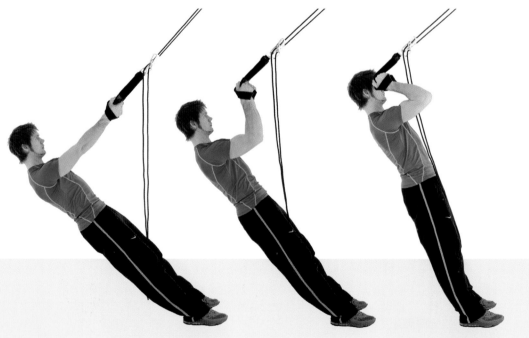

3.16 One arm bicep curl

Stand sideways holding on to one sling and lean back on your extended arm. Your upper arm should be in a fixed position while performing the movement. With the palm facing upward, bend the elbow to pull yourself up to a standing position. Hold for a second, then return to starting position.

Expert advice: Keeping the upper arm stationary requires actively pushing the arm upward while you are performing the exercise. To get a feel for the correct position for the arm, try the correct start and end positions before attempting the exercise.

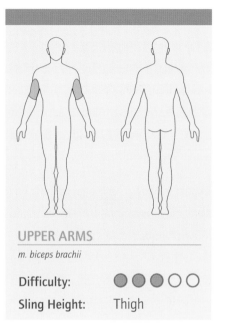

UPPER ARMS

m. biceps brachii

Difficulty: ●●●○○

Sling Height: Thigh

79

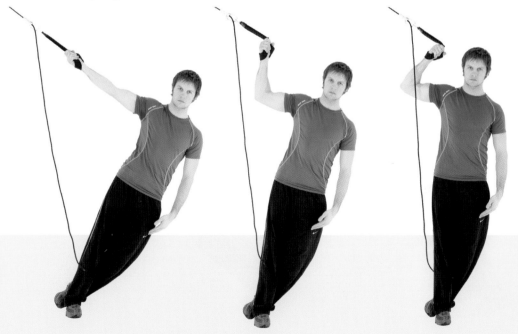

3.17 Triceps press

Start in the forward position. Lean forward on extended arms, supported by the slings. Thumbs should be facing toward you. Keep the upper arms fixed while you bend the elbows, letting the body sink forward. Hold and return when your hands are by your ears.

Expert advice: The higher you lift your arms over your head, the more triceps muscle you exercise.

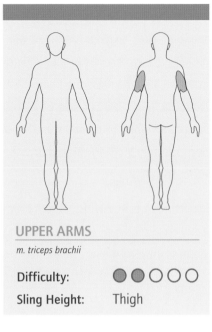

UPPER ARMS

m. triceps brachii

Difficulty: ●●○○○

Sling Height: Thigh

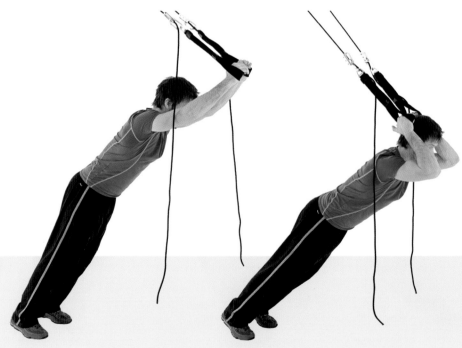

3.18 One arm triceps press

Stand sideways and hold on to a sling. Lean toward the sling supported on one arm, thumb facing the ceiling. Keeping your upper arm in a fixed position, bend the elbow and lean farther into the sling. Hold for a second, and then return by pushing off and straightening the elbow.

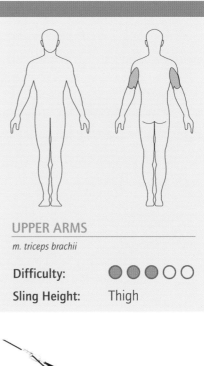

UPPER ARMS

m. triceps brachii

Difficulty: ●●●○○

Sling Height: Thigh

81

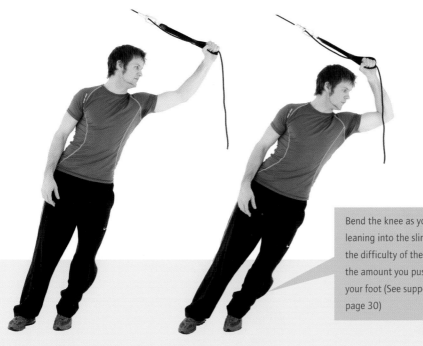

Bend the knee as you are leaning into the sling. Adjust the difficulty of the exercise by the amount you push off with your foot (See supporting foot, page 30)

3.19 Incline push-ups

Start in the forward position. Lean forward by bending the elbows. Press back to starting position and repeat.

Expert advice: For beginners, concentrate on keeping the slings steady in your hands. Hold your hands higher than the elbows to avoid undue friction from the ropes.

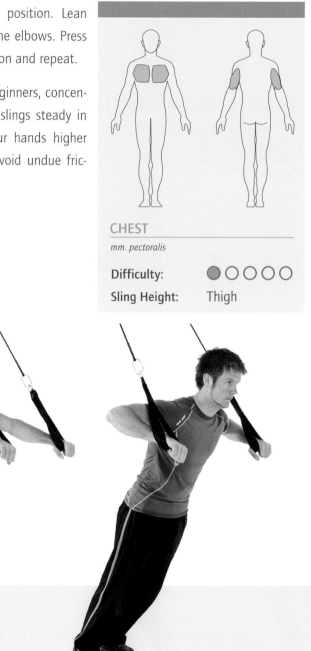

CHEST

mm. pectoralis

Difficulty: ●○○○○

Sling Height: Thigh

3.20 Push-ups

Perform like incline push-ups (exercise 3.19).

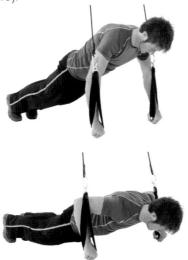

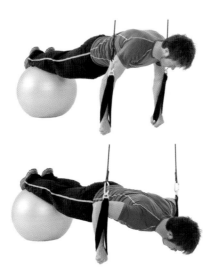

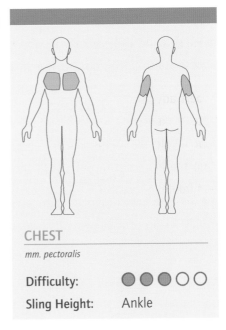

CHEST

mm. pectoralis

Difficulty: ●●●○○

Sling Height: Ankle

83

3.21 Push-ups on a fitness ball

Perform like incline push-ups (exercise 3.19), but with feet wide and resting on a fitness ball.

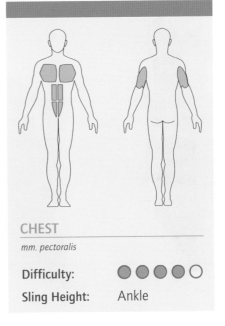

CHEST

mm. pectoralis

Difficulty: ●●●●○

Sling Height: Ankle

3.22 Supported dips

Stand with one hand in each sling, arms straight with shoulders above hands. Feet should be crossed and resting on the floor. Lower body toward the floor by bending at the elbows. When a stretch is felt in chest or shoulders, push body up until arms are straight. Use your feet to help reduce the amount of weight you lift, and avoid locking your elbows when arms are straight.

Expert advice: If your hand grip gets uncomfortable, try placing your fists inside the slings.

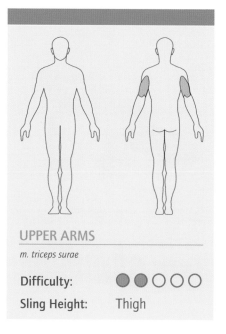

UPPER ARMS

m. triceps surae

Difficulty:	●●○○○
Sling Height:	Thigh

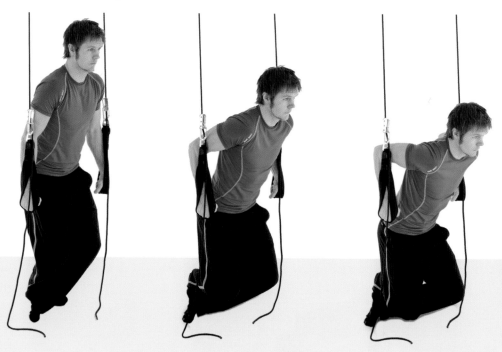

3.23 Dips

Hoist up into the slings on straight arms, shoulders above hands. Lower your body by bending at the elbows. When a stretch is felt in chest or shoulders, push body up until arms are straight. Avoid locking the elbows when your arms are straight.

Expert advice: If your hand grip gets uncomfortable, try placing your fists inside the slings.

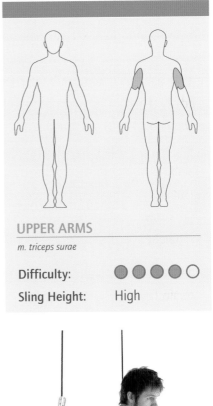

UPPER ARMS

m. triceps surae

Difficulty:	●●●●○
Sling Height:	High

85

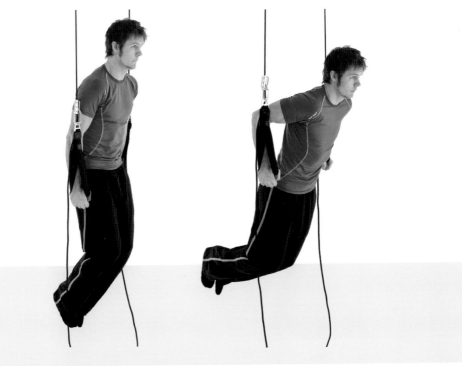

3.24 Pull-ups

Reach and grasp the slings with a wide overhand grip. Lift your feet off the ground. Crossing is optional. Using your arms, lift your body until the chin is the same height as your hands. Lower body until arms are straight.

Expert advice: Avoid locking the elbows when the arms are straight by keeping ready tension in the biceps and shoulders.

ARMS & UPPER BACK

m. latissimus, m. biceps brachii

Difficulty: ●●●○○

Sling Height: High

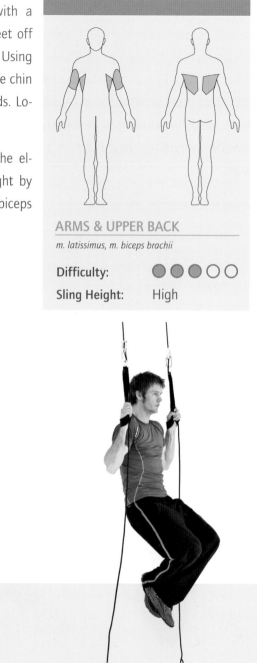

3.25 Incline pull-ups to triceps press

Begin in the backward position. Keep shoulders low, chest pushed forward. Lift yourself up by pulling the elbows down and out to the side. Stop when the elbows are at 90 degrees to the arms. Hold the elbows still and push forward by pressing your hands outward.

Release back down and repeat.

Expert advice: Hold the slings as you would hold a rope, palms facing downward. Keep your wrists firm while pushing your hands outward.

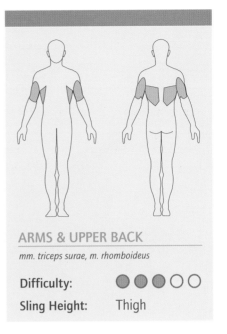

ARMS & UPPER BACK

mm. triceps surae, m. rhomboideus

Difficulty: ●●●○○

Sling Height: Thigh

87

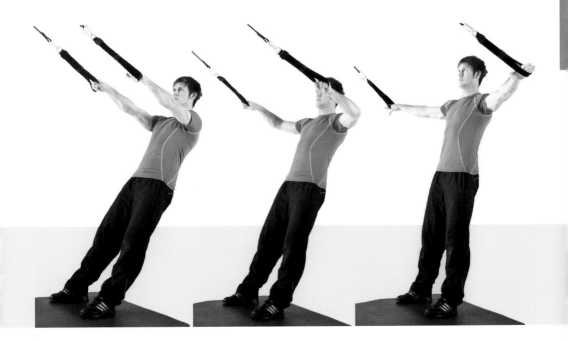

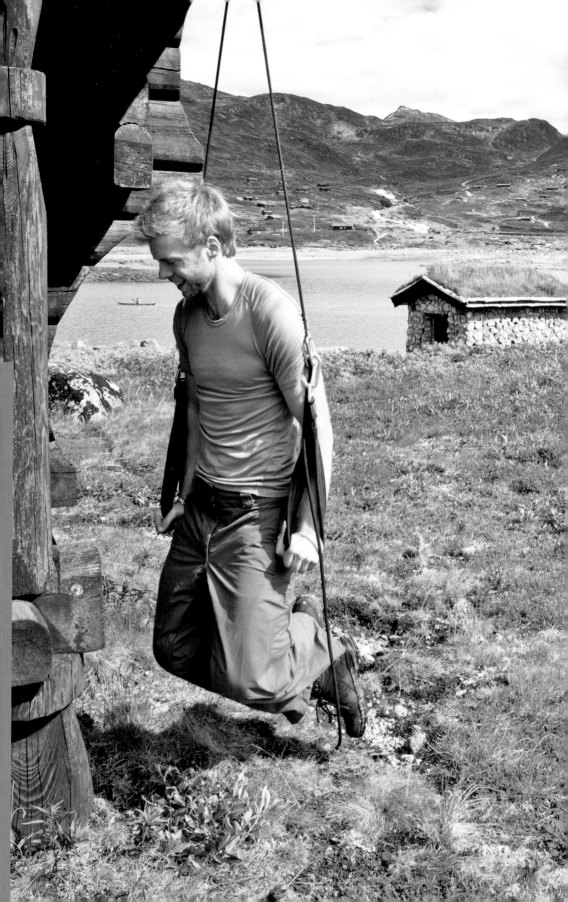

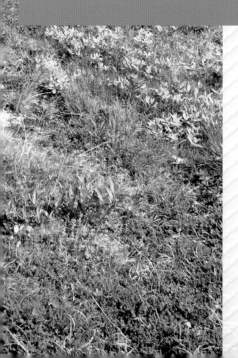
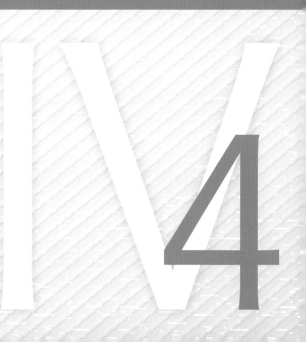

PART **IV**

CHAPTER 4

EXERCISES
CORE

IV 4

Chapter 4

CORE

4.1 Forward lean

Stand a foot or two in front of the slings. Lean forward with elbows in slings, supporting your body on extended arms. The arms should be at 90 degrees to the body. Keep the back in a neutral spine position. Keep your body in a straight line – it's easy to cheat by bending at the hips.

When exercising you should feel the abs working. Hold the position for 10 seconds.

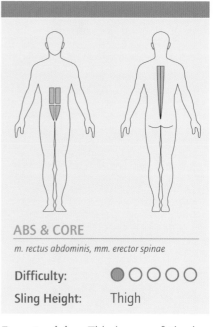

ABS & CORE

m. rectus abdominis, mm. erector spinae

Difficulty: ●○○○○

Sling Height: Thigh

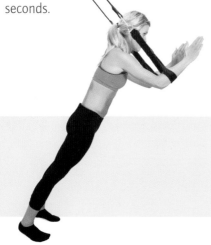

Expert advice: This is one of the basic positions. You should master this position first, as many other exercises begin in this way. If you start to feel strain, tiredness or pain in the lower back – stop immediately. Return to start. Make the exercise easier and find your neutral spine position.

4.2   Knees off the ground

Begin on all fours, hands in slings. Get on your toes and lift your knees off the floor. Hold the position for 30 seconds, then lower knees to the floor.

Expert advice: This exercise works the abdominals statically in a different position than the usual plank. The exercise looks easier than it is!

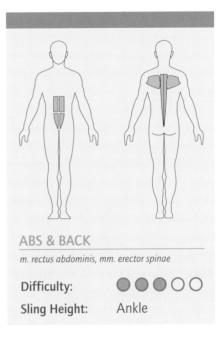

ABS & BACK
m. rectus abdominis, mm. erector spinae

Difficulty: ●●●○○

Sling Height: Ankle

91

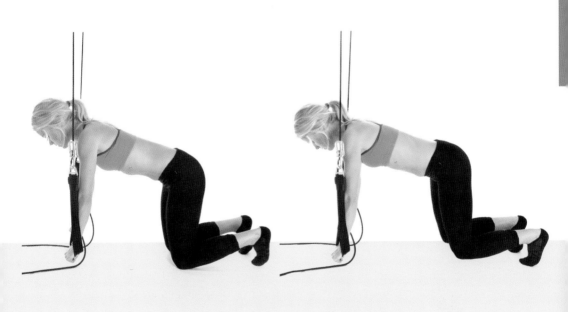

4.3   The plank

Lie face down, one foot in each sling and knees and elbows resting on the floor. Support yourself on your forearms, tighten your abs and lift your knees off the floor. Body should be level from head to toe. Forearms and feet should carry equal weight.

Hold for 30 seconds or move on to the next pages to see different dynamic variations of the plank.

Expert advice: This exercise is the basis for all the best core exercises. Do this exercise well and you'll progress faster through all sling exercises.

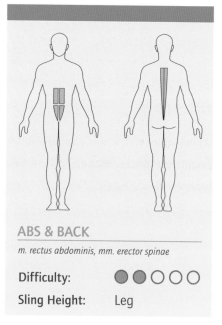

ABS & BACK

m. rectus abdominis, mm. erector spinae

Difficulty: ●●○○○

Sling Height: Leg

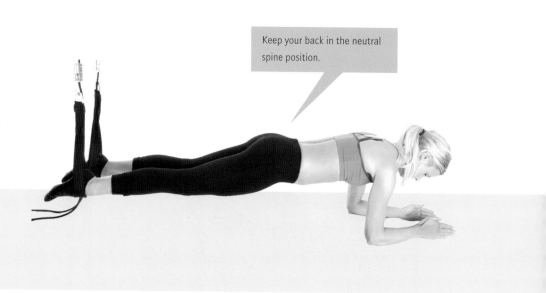

Keep your back in the neutral spine position.

4.4 Sling cycling

Start in plank position (exercise 4.3). Alternately draw your knees up toward your elbows. The exercise should flow dynamically with a cycle-like movement of the legs.

Expert advice: Try to keep the same weight on each leg as you move through the exercise. This will keep your body from rotating back and forth.

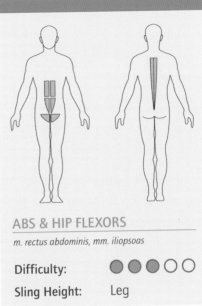

ABS & HIP FLEXORS

m. rectus abdominis, mm. iliopsoas

Difficulty: ●●●○○
Sling Height: Leg

93

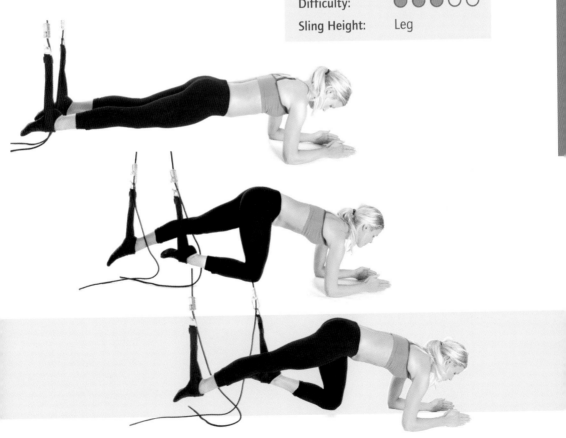

4.5   Omega

Start in plank position (exercise 4.3). Draw your knees up to your elbows. Hold for one second before returning to plank position.

Expert advice: Avoid sagging down to the floor when tired; keep the neutral spine position. Think this is too easy? Try Omega with just one foot in a sling. Keep the unsupported leg at the same height and do the exercise without rotating your body.

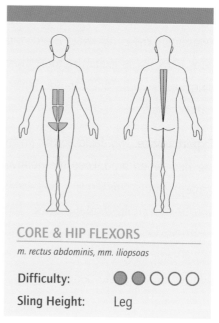

CORE & HIP FLEXORS

m. rectus abdominis, mm. iliopsoas

Difficulty: ●●○○○
Sling Height: Leg

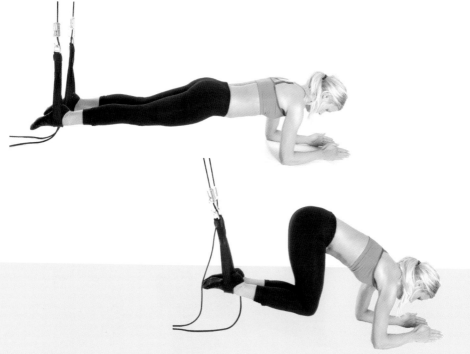

4.6   Sideways omega

Start in plank position (exercise 4.3). Draw your knees up and toward one side. Hold for a second before returning to plank position. Repeat, alternating sides.

Expert advice: Avoid sagging down to the floor when tired, keep the neutral spine position. Think this is too easy? Try the Sidecrunch with just one foot in a sling. Keep the unsupported leg at the same height and do the exercise without rotating your body.

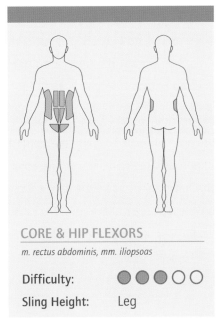

CORE & HIP FLEXORS

m. rectus abdominis, mm. iliopsoas

Difficulty: ●●●○○

Sling Height: Leg

95

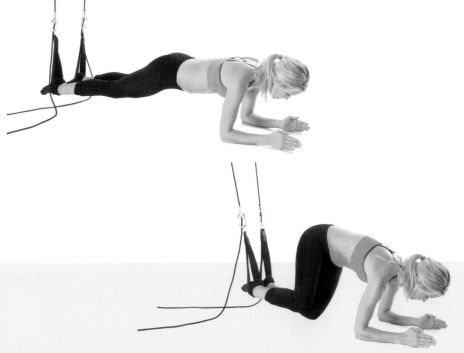

4.7   Twisted plank

Start in plank position (exercise 4.3). Shift your weight to one forearm, lift the other arm off the floor and rotate your body to a side plank. Hold for a second, return to plank position and repeat, alternating sides.

Expert advice: If you feel unsure about this exercise, try it first with your feet on the floor.

OBLIQUES

mm. obliquus, m. rectus abdominis

Difficulty: ●●○○○

Sling Height: Leg

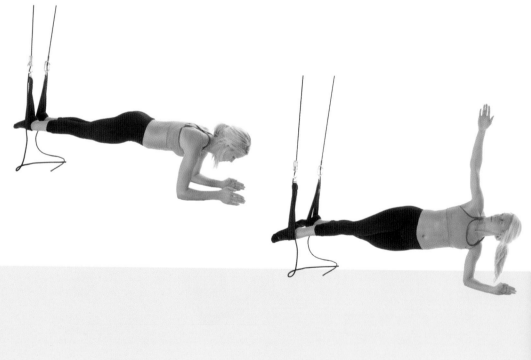

4.8 Delta

Start in plank position (exercise 4.3). Pike your hips up while drawing your feet toward you. Keep your legs straight, knees extended, throughout the movement.

Expert advice: Look down toward your feet as you pull your feet toward you. This helps bring the whole body into the movement.

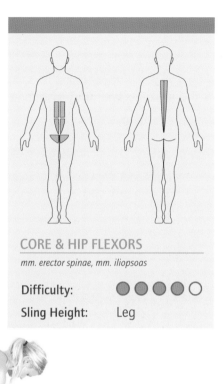

CORE & HIP FLEXORS

mm. erector spinae, mm. iliopsoas

Difficulty: ●●●●○

Sling Height: Leg

4.9 Body saw

Start in plank position (exercise 4.3). Push off with your forearms to bring your body backward. Keep your back in the neutral spine position throughout the exercise.

Expert advice: To increase difficulty you may do the exercise on straight arms.

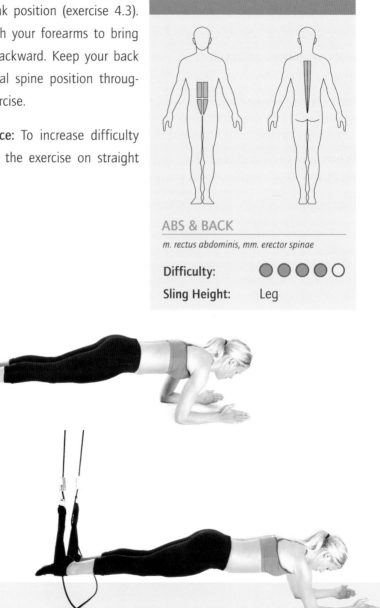

ABS & BACK

m. rectus abdominis, mm. erector spinae

Difficulty: ●●●●○

Sling Height: Leg

4.10 Side plank

Lie sideways on the floor with your feet in a wide sling. With the elbow in line with the shoulders, lift your hips off the floor and straighten your back. Hold for 30 seconds before lowering hips to the floor.

Expert advice: This is the basic static exercise for the obliques, the muscles shaping your waistline. The next page will describe the dynamic side plank.

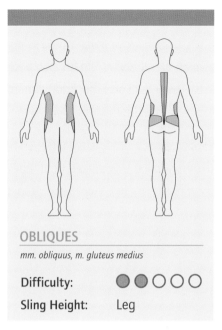

OBLIQUES

mm. obliquus, m. gluteus medius

Difficulty: ●●○○○

Sling Height: Leg

99

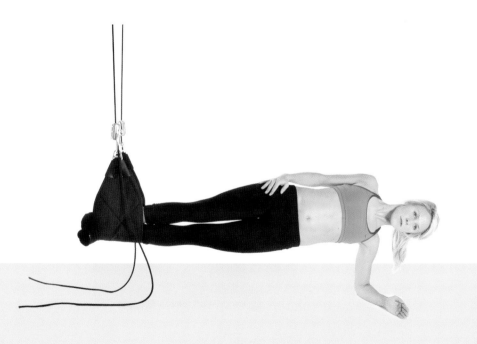

4.11 Dynamic side plank

Start in side plank position (exercise 4.10). Lift your hips toward the ceiling, as high as you can. Hold for a second, then lower hips to the floor. Before touching the floor, start another repetition.

Expert advice: Make sure your body is straight. No twisting. Keep proper form!

OBLIQUES

mm. obliquus, m. gluteus medius

Difficulty: ●●●○○

Sling Height: Leg

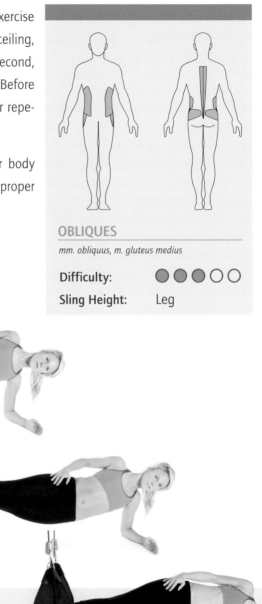

4.12 Supine plank

Lie on your back, feet in slings. Lift your hips by pressing feet downward. The body should be straight, your back in the neutral spine position.

Static exercise: Hold for 30 seconds, then lower hips to the floor.

Dynamic exercise: Start in supine plank position. Lower hips close to the floor, then lift your hips back to starting position. Repeat.

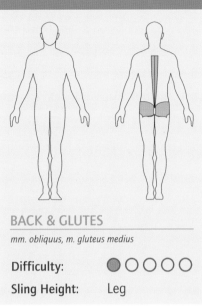

BACK & GLUTES

mm. obliquus, m. gluteus medius

Difficulty: ●○○○○

Sling Height: Leg

101

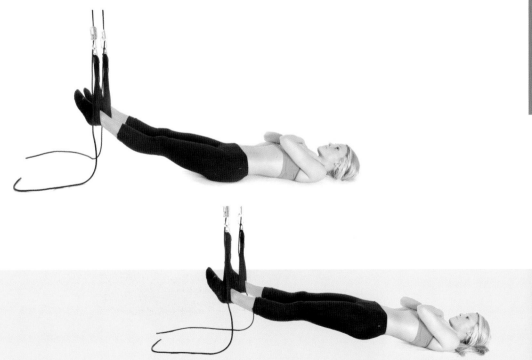

4.13 One leg supine plank

Begin in supine plank (exercise 4.12). Keep only one leg in a sling, the other leg unsupported but held at the same height. Lift the hips and hold your body straight. Keep your back in the neutral spine position; work the obliques to keep your body from rotating.

Variation: If you want to increase difficulty, you may try the One Leg Extended Reverse Plank. Starting in the position described above, move the free leg out to the side. Hold for a second and return parallel to the leg in the sling.

BACK & HAMSTRINGS

mm. erector spinae, m. semitendinosus, m. semimembranosus, m. biceps femoris

Difficulty: ●●●○○

Sling Height: Leg

4.14 Supine plank rotation

Start in supine plank with one leg in a sling (exercise 4.12). From this position, rotate your body toward the floor. Rotate until almost touching the floor then turn back to starting position. Rotate through the hips and legs, keeping the back in a neutral spine position.

Expert advice: Elite soccer players use this exercise. It simulates the demands on the stabilizing muscles at the moment of kicking the ball.

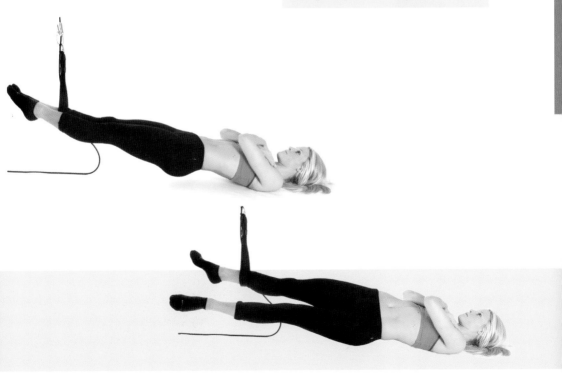

OBLIQUES & HAMSTRINGS

mm. erector spinae, m. semitendinosus, m. semimembranosus, m. biceps femoris

Difficulty: ●●●○○

Sling Height: Leg

103

4.15 Sling bridge

Lie on your back with feet in the sling trainer. Keep knees at a 90 degree angle and lift the hips. Hold for a second before lowering hips to the floor. Repeat.

GLUTES & BACK

mm. gluteus, mm. erector spinae

Difficulty: ●●○○○

Sling Height: Ankle

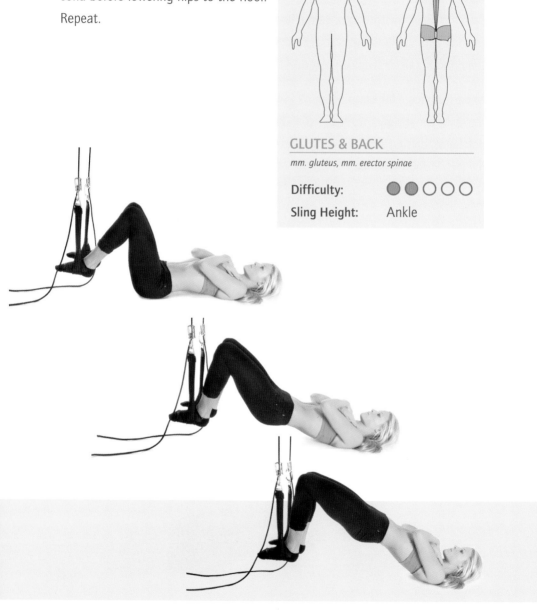

4.16 Reverse sling cycling

Start in a sling bridge (exercise 4.15). Alternately, draw the legs toward you. Move smoothly in a cycle-like fashion.

Expert advice: Concentrate on keeping equal weight on each leg throughout the movement.

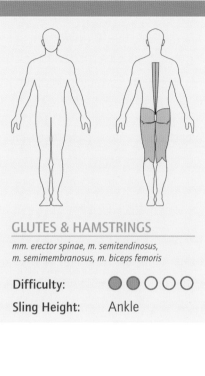

GLUTES & HAMSTRINGS

mm. erector spinae, m. semitendinosus, m. semimembranosus, m. biceps femoris

Difficulty: ●●○○○

Sling Height: Ankle

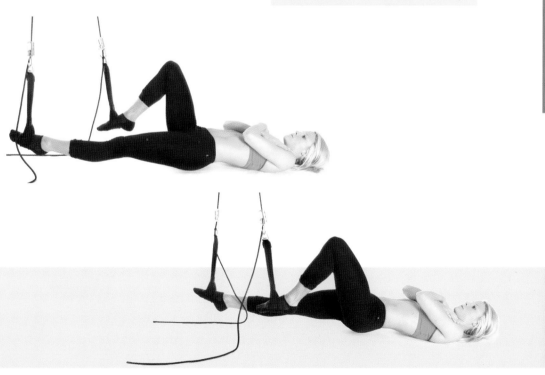

4.17 Leg lifts

Lie on your back, one hand in each sling. Using slings for support, tighten abs and lift your legs off the floor. Flex feet straight up in the air and then lower slowly to the ground. Repeat.

Expert advice: It is easy to overarch your back when lifting or lowering your legs. Make sure to keep your back in the neutral spine position.

Variation: Instead of straight up and down, try moving your feet in a figure eight pattern to activate the obliques.

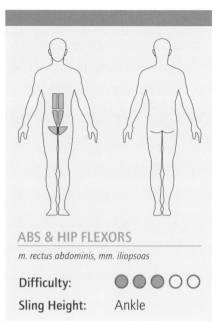

ABS & HIP FLEXORS

m. rectus abdominis, mm. iliopsoas

Difficulty: ●●●○○
Sling Height: Ankle

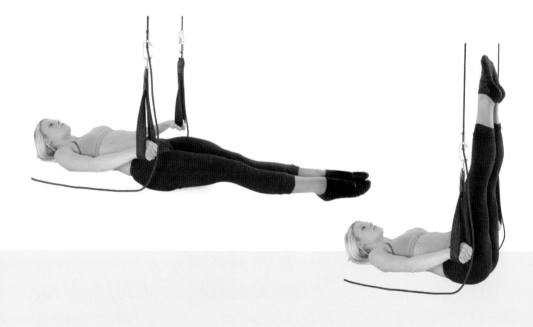

4.18 Wide sling obliques

Lie sideways in a wide sling. Find your balance with the waist supported by the sling. Hands behind your head, lower the upper body sideways toward the floor. Then raise the upper body, activating the oblique abdominals.

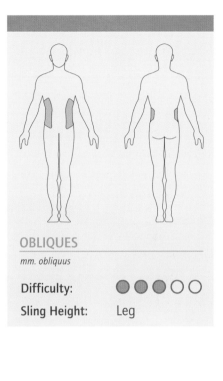

OBLIQUES

mm. obliquus

Difficulty: ●●●○○

Sling Height: Leg

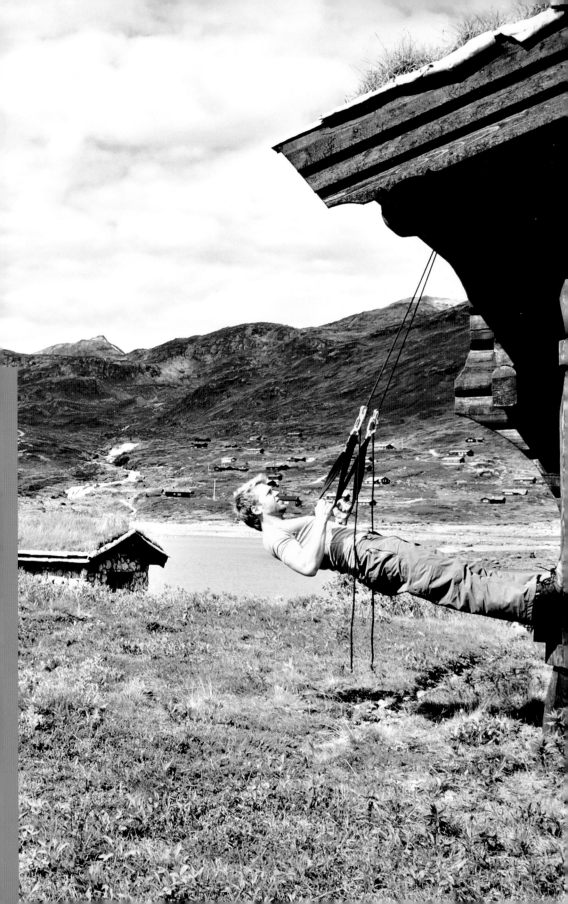

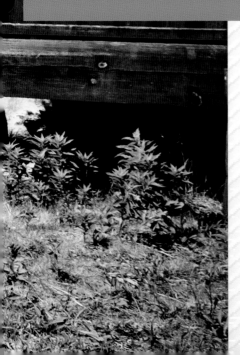
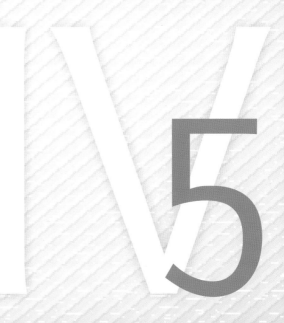

PART IV

CHAPTER 5

EXERCISES
EXTREME SLING TRAINING

IV

IV 5

Chapter 5

EXTREME SLING TRAINING

5.1 Extreme plank

Start with your knees in a wide sling. Lean forward until you are in a plank position (exercise 4.3), arms straight. Walk backward on your hands until your body is at 45 degrees to the floor. Push your body backward while holding your arms straight. Return to the plank position and then repeat.

Expert advice: Keep your lower back in a neutral position throughout the movement. For a harder exercise, move the wide sling toward your feet.

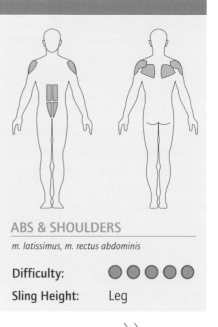

ABS & SHOULDERS

m. latissimus, m. rectus abdominis

Difficulty: ●●●●●

Sling Height: Leg

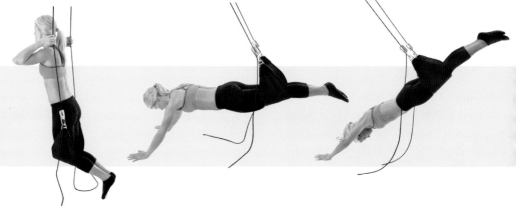

5.2 Incline handstand press

Start in an Extreme plank (exercise 5.1). Bend your elbows until your head touches the floor, then push back to straight elbows.

Expert advice: Keep your lower back in a neutral position throughout the movement. For a harder exercise, move the wide sling towards your feet.

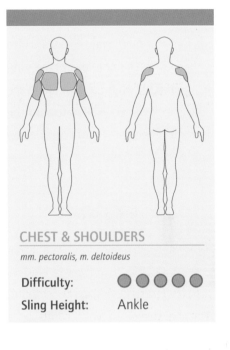

CHEST & SHOULDERS

mm. pectoralis, m. deltoideus

Difficulty: ●●●●●

Sling Height: Ankle

111

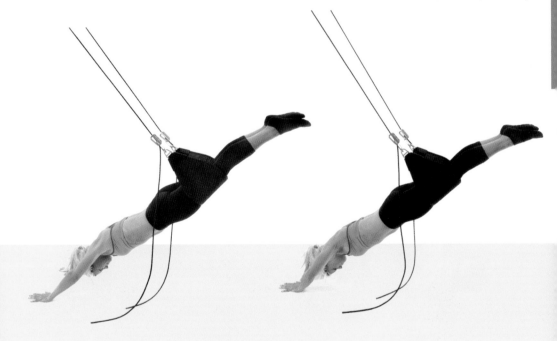

5.3 Handstand press

Start in plank position, but with only one foot in a sling. Walk backward into a handstand. The one foot in the sling helps you keep your balance. Bend the elbows to lower your body toward the floor. Push back to straight arms. Keep your back in a neutral spine position, legs straight.

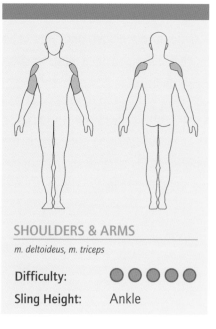

SHOULDERS & ARMS

m. deltoideus, m. triceps

Difficulty:	●●●●●
Sling Height:	Ankle

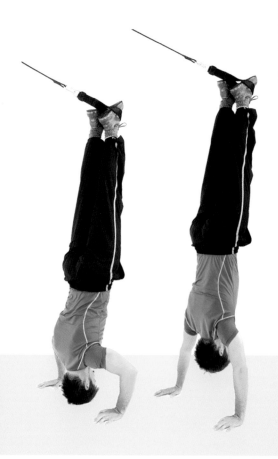

5.4   Twisted side plank

Start in a side plank (exercise 4.10) with the free arm pointing to the ceiling. Tighten the abs, lift your hips and cross the free arm below and behind you. Hold for a second and then return to starting position.

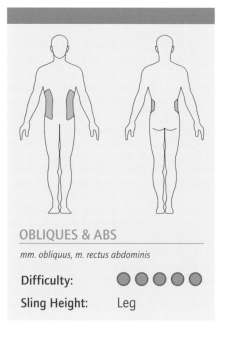

OBLIQUES & ABS

mm. obliquus, m. rectus abdominis

Difficulty: ●●●●●
Sling Height: Leg

113

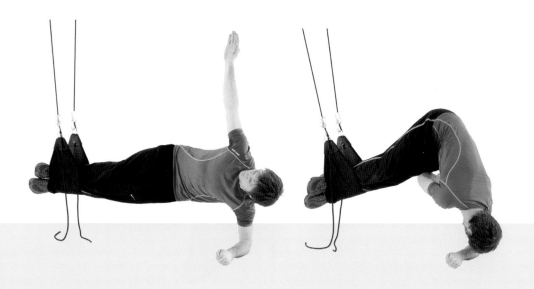

5.5. One hand one foot omega

Start in plank position (exercise 4.1), but with only one foot in the sling and one hand for support. Draw your knees up toward your elbows. Hold for one second before returning to plank position. Repeat.

Expert advice: Keep the unsupported leg at the same height and do the exercise without rotating your body.

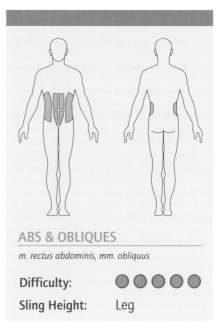

ABS & OBLIQUES

m. rectus abdominis, mm. obliquus

Difficulty: ●●●●●
Sling Height: Leg

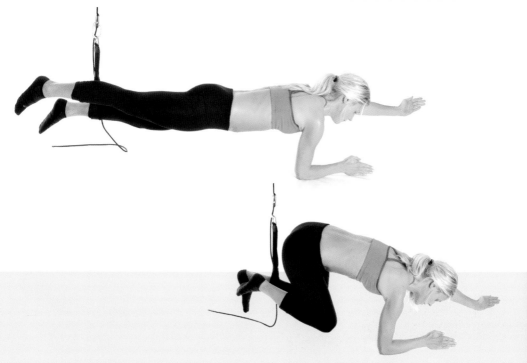

5.6 Double poling plank

Start in plank position (exercise 4.3). The elbows should be in line with the shoulders, hands pointing forward. Lean backward before pushing forward, palms to the floor, lifting yourself on to straight arms.

Expert advice: Make the exercise easier by doing a body saw (exercise 4.9). The added speed and momentum will make it easier to lift yourself on to straight arms.

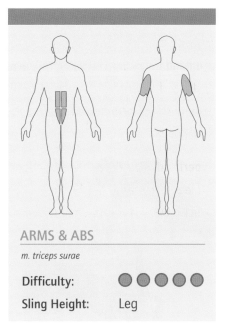

ARMS & ABS

m. triceps surae

Difficulty: ● ● ● ● ●

Sling Height: Leg

115

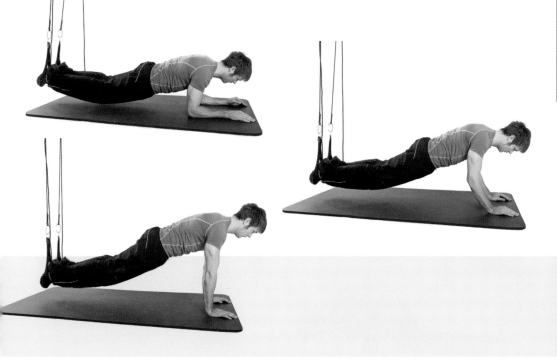

5.7 One arm supported push-up

Start with one hand in a sling, the other on the floor. The sling is only for support to ease into learning one arm push-ups. Perform the exercise like regular push-ups (exercise 3.20).

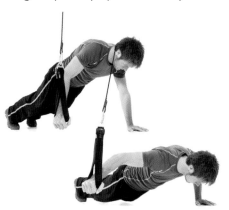

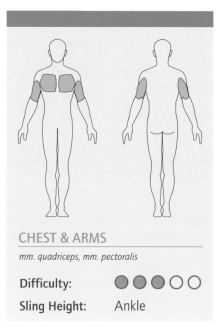

CHEST & ARMS

mm. quadriceps, mm. pectoralis

Difficulty: ●●●○○

Sling Height: Ankle

5.8 One arm sling push-ups

With one arm in a sling and the other arm resting on your back, lower your body by bending at the elbow. Raise yourself back to starting position by straightening the arm.

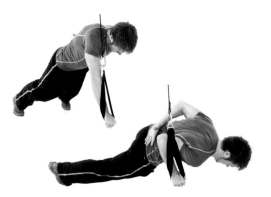

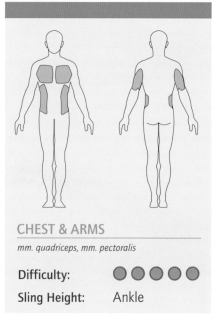

CHEST & ARMS

mm. quadriceps, mm. pectoralis

Difficulty: ●●●●●

Sling Height: Ankle

5.9   Straddle sit to half flair

Begin in a push-up position with one foot in a sling. Swing your feet to the left and forward. Lift your left arm to let the right leg come through and point forward. End up with feet hovering over the floor, supported by your arms. Hold this position and ignore the envious looks from people around you. Then return to starting position by lifting your left arm and swinging your legs out and behind you. Repeat and turn to the other side.

Expert advice: Credit to Linzi Co for this exercise. Check out our blog for link to her YouTubevideos (www.slingexercises.com/linzi).

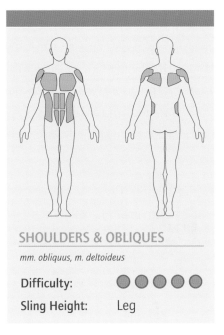

SHOULDERS & OBLIQUES

mm. obliquus, m. deltoideus

Difficulty: ⬤⬤⬤⬤⬤

Sling Height: Leg

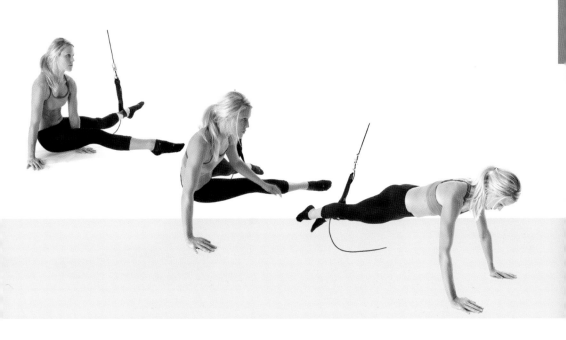

5.10 Wide sling leg lifts

Lie down in the wide sling. Lift your legs and find your balance with the lower back supported by the sling. Tighten abs and lift your legs off the floor. Point feet straight up in the air and then lower slowly until horizontal. Repeat.

Expert advice: It is easy to over arch your back when lifting or lowering your legs. Make sure to keep your back in the neutral spine position.

Variation: Instead of straight up and down, try moving your feet in a figure eight pattern to activate the obliques.

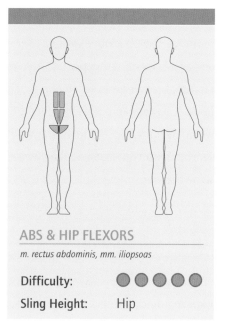

ABS & HIP FLEXORS
m. rectus abdominis, mm. iliopsoas

Difficulty: ●●●●●
Sling Height: Hip

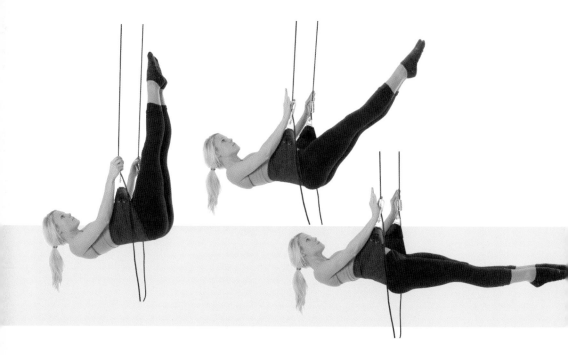

5.11 Extreme swing

Place the wide sling right above your buttocks. Lean backward into the sling and swing forward. Keep your feet up, abs engaged as you swing back and forth. It is easy to overarch your back when swinging back and forth. Make sure to keep your back in the neutral spine position.

Expert Advice: How you place the wide sling makes all the difference. When you place the sling above the upper part of the buttocks, you will need extreme core control to avoid overarching your back.

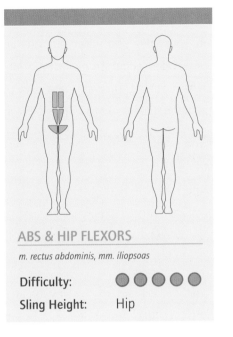

ABS & HIP FLEXORS

m. rectus abdominis, mm. iliopsoas

Difficulty: ● ● ● ● ●

Sling Height: Hip

119

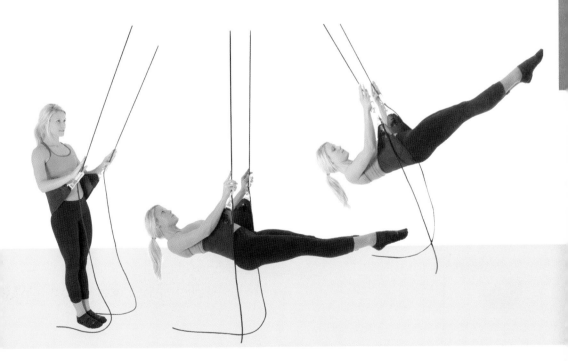

5.12 Hanging leg raises

With both hands, grab on to the slings. Lift your body and raise your legs up toward the ceiling. From this position, lower legs until they are parallel with the floor. Repeat.

Expert advice: Beginners, you may start by doing the exercise with knees bent.

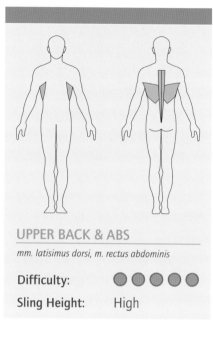

UPPER BACK & ABS

mm. latisimus dorsi, m. rectus abdominis

Difficulty: ●●●●●
Sling Height: High

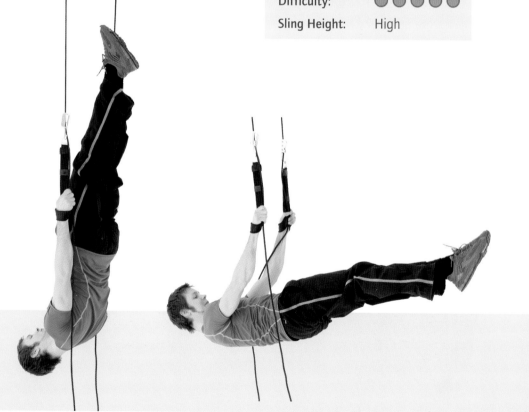

5.13 V-ups

Hang by your arms in the sling trainer. Lift your legs up in front of you, forming a V-shape with your body. From this position, use your arms to pull yourself up until your chin reaches sling height. Lower back down and repeat.

UPPER BACK & ARMS

m. latissimus dorsi, m. biceps brachii

Difficulty: ● ● ● ● ●

Sling Height: High

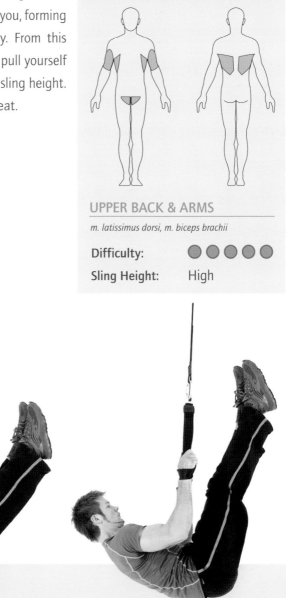

5.14 Hanging and turning

With both hands, grab on to the slings. Lift your body parallel to the floor and raise your legs up toward the ceiling. From this position, lower legs to the side until parallel with the floor. Return and repeat to the other side.

Expert advice: Beginners, you may start by doing the exercise with knees bent.

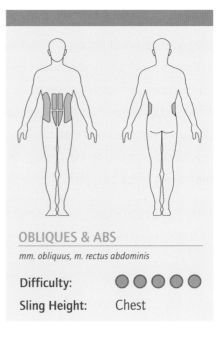

OBLIQUES & ABS

mm. obliquus, m. rectus abdominis

Difficulty: ⬤⬤⬤⬤⬤

Sling Height: Chest

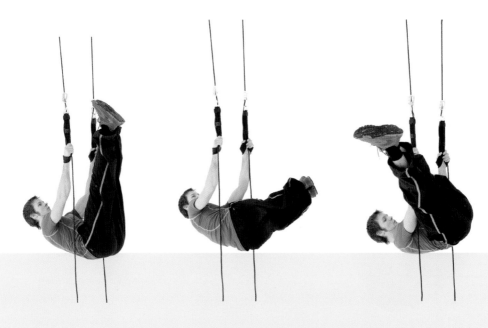

5.15 Sling handstands

Hoist yourself up on straight arms in the slings. Lift your legs up in front of you until parallel with the floor. From this position, bend the elbows and lean forward. Continue leaning forward until you are perpendicular with the floor, legs flexed pointing to the ceiling. Return slowly to starting position.

Expert advice: To make the exercise harder, keep your arms straight from start to finish.

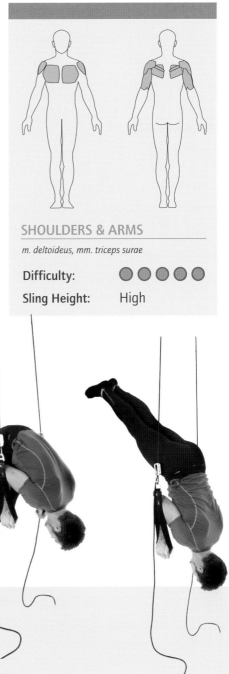

SHOULDERS & ARMS

m. deltoideus, mm. triceps surae

Difficulty: ●●●●●

Sling Height: High

123

5.16 Twisted push-ups

Begin in plank position, straight arms in the slings. Shift your body weight to one arm and lift the other toward the ceiling. Hold for a second and return to starting position. Do a push-up (exercise 3.20) then repeat the move to the opposite side.

Expert advice: This exercise will build shoulder stability and strength. If you are a beginner, first try the exercise with hands on the floor.

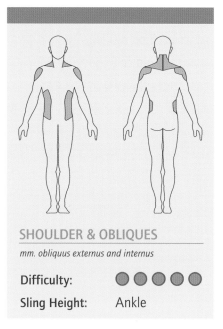

SHOULDER & OBLIQUES

mm. obliquus externus and internus

Difficulty: ⬤⬤⬤⬤⬤

Sling Height: Ankle

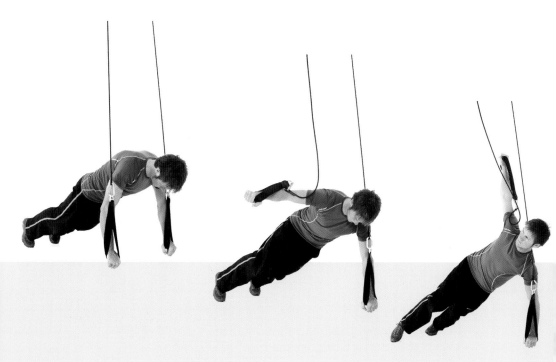

5.17 The egg

Begin lying on your back, feet in slings. Pull yourself up by your legs as high as you can. Hold for a second and then lower yourself to the floor. Repeat.

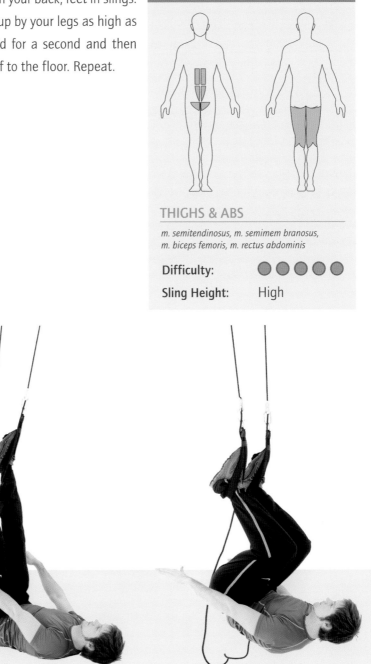

THIGHS & ABS

m. semitendinosus, m. semimem branosus, m. biceps femoris, m. rectus abdominis

Difficulty: ●●●●●

Sling Height: High

125

5.18 Hanging sit-ups

Fasten your feet in the slings. You should hang freely without touching the ground. Pull your upper body toward your knees. Release then lower down in a controlled manner. Repeat.

Expert advice: You may perform this exercise as a straight sit up or with elbow to opposite knee to work the obliques (as shown in the second photo).

Warning! Do not hang in the slings without anyone nearby! You may not be able to get back down!

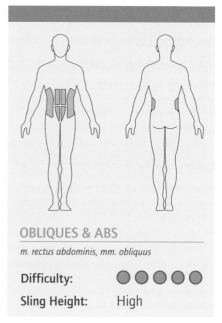

OBLIQUES & ABS

m. rectus abdominis, mm. obliquus

Difficulty: ● ● ● ● ●

Sling Height: High

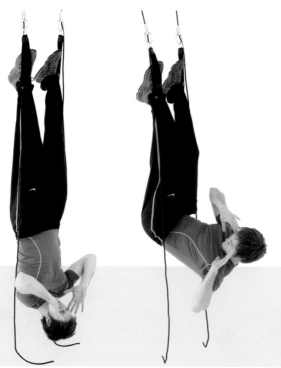

5.19 Sling squat

Place one foot in each sling and stand up. Feet should be supported by slings, not touching the floor. Keep your feet balanced as you bend your knees. Hold for a second and then straighten the legs.

Expert advice: For extra support, you may hold on to the ropes with your hands. This makes the exercise easier.

THIGHS & ABS

m. semitendinosus, m. semimem branosus, m. biceps femoris, m. rectus abdominis

Difficulty: ● ● ● ● ●

Sling Height: Ankle

127

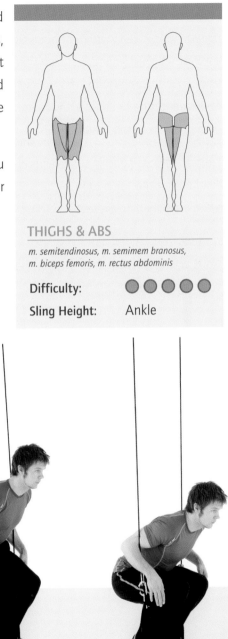

5.20 Typewriter pull-ups

Grab the slings and cross your feet, body hanging freely off the floor. Pull yourself up until your chin is at sling height. From this position, pull yourself from side to side by shifting the weight from one arm to the other.

Expert advice: When you start losing height, it's time for a break! This is a great rock-climbing exercise.

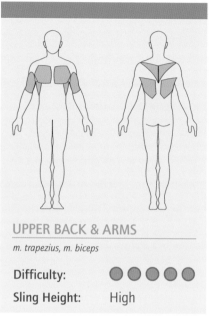

UPPER BACK & ARMS

m. trapezius, m. biceps

Difficulty: ●●●●●
Sling Height: High

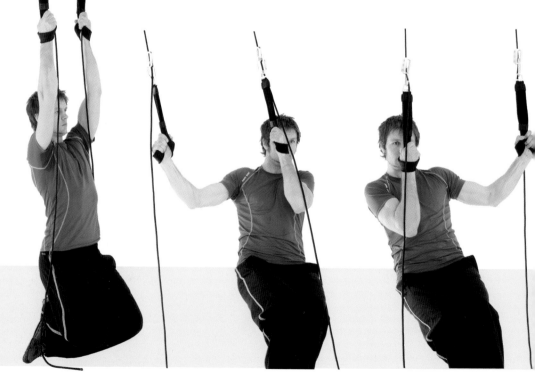

5.21 Supported one hand pull-up

Adjust the slings so that one is 11 inches (30 cm) higher than the other. Grab the slings and cross your feet, body hanging freely off the floor. Start with the highest arm hanging straight. Pull yourself up with the highest arm and push off with the lower-hanging arm. Keep the lower arms' elbow close to your body throughout the movement.

Expert advice: This is the last step before the fabled one hand pull-up! You may have to adjust the height between the two slings to find the right height for you.

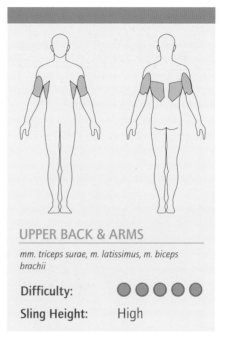

UPPER BACK & ARMS

mm. triceps surae, m. latissimus, m. biceps brachii

Difficulty: ⬤⬤⬤⬤⬤

Sling Height: High

129

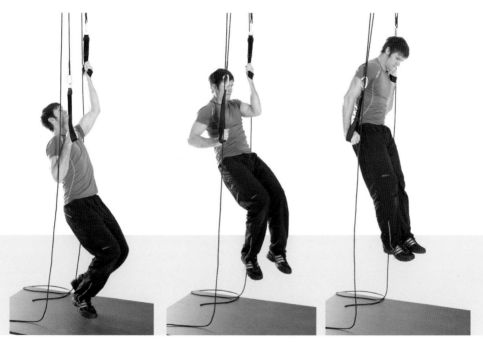

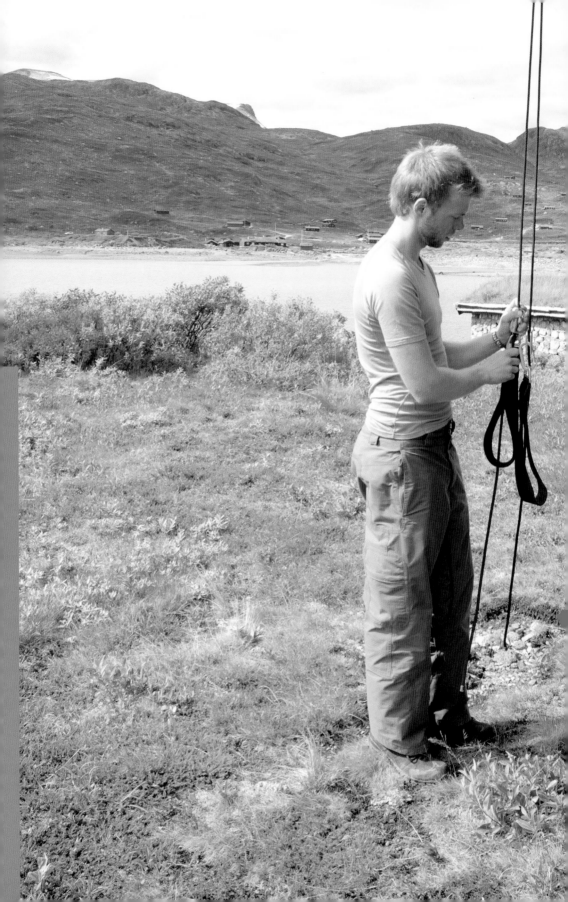

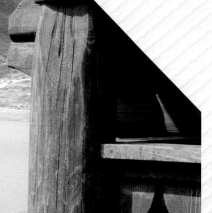
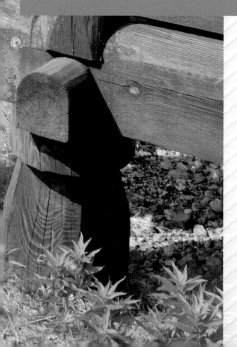
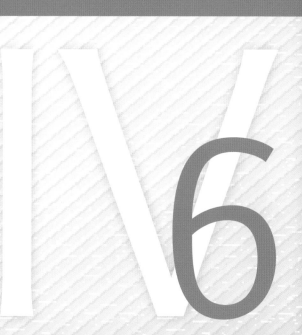

PART IV

CHAPTER 6

EXERCISES
STRETCHING
AND RELAXATION

IV

6

Chapter 6

STRETCHING AND RELAXATION

6.1 Upper back mobilization

Sit on a fitness ball or on the edge of a chair, right under the point of sling attachment. Cross your arms and place them in a wide sling. Rest your head in your arms and lean forward. Let your chest drop to the floor and sink into the sling. You should feel the stretch in the upper back and chest.

Expert advice: If your job involves sitting in front of the computer, you may have felt stiffness and soreness of the

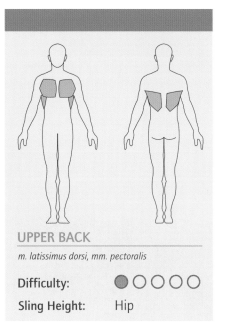

UPPER BACK

m. latissimus dorsi, mm. pectoralis

Difficulty: ● ○ ○ ○ ○

Sling Height: Hip

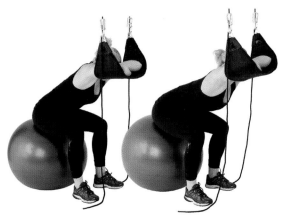

upper back after long work hours. This exercise will help you regain flexibility and relax stiff muscles.

Remember that the movement should be in your upper back, not in your shoulders.

6.2 Lateral back stretch

Start in the position of upper back mobilization (exercise 6.1). Lean over to one side until you feel a stretch along the opposite side of the body. Hold the stretch for 30 seconds, and then move to the other side.

Expert advice: For relaxation, you may move dynamically. Relax your muscles and float from side to side without pause.

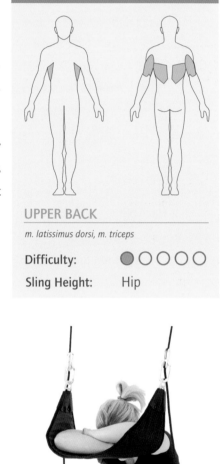

UPPER BACK

m. latissimus dorsi, m. triceps

Difficulty: ●○○○○

Sling Height: Hip

133

6.3   Pectoralis stretch

Cross the ropes so the left sling is in your right hand and vice versa. Stretch your arms out to each side and push your chest up. Walk slowly forward until you feel a stretch across your chest. Adjust the height of your arms to stretch different parts of your chest muscle.

Expert advice: If you feel a stretch in your shoulders, not your chest, try rotating your arms outward. Palms should be facing forward throughout the movement

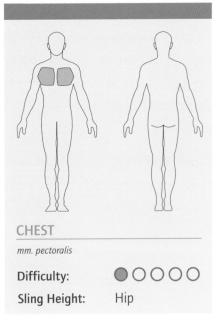

CHEST

mm. pectoralis

Difficulty: ●○○○○

Sling Height: Hip

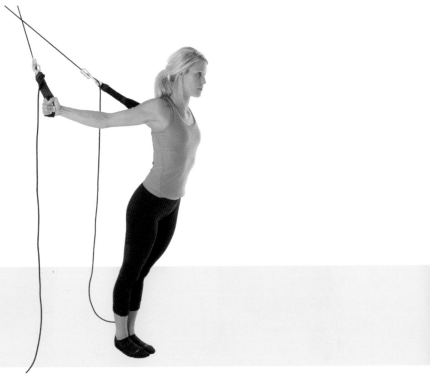

6.4   Latissimus stretch

Begin with one sling in each hand. Lift one arm as high as you can and lean over to the opposite side. You should feel a stretch along the side of your upper body.

UPPER BACK

m. lattissimus

Difficulty: ●○○○○

Sling Height: Hip

135

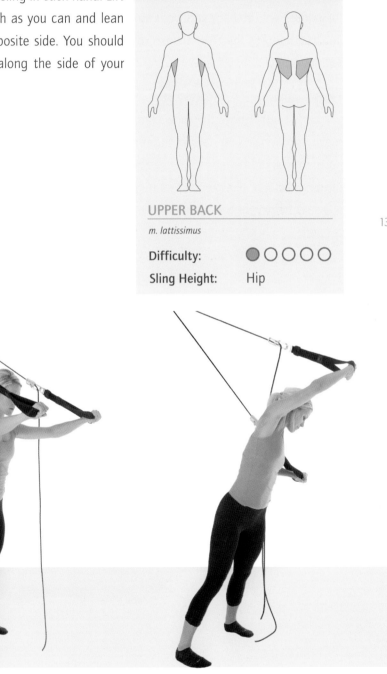

6.5 Back mobilization

Place the wide sling right above the lumbar spine. Lean back until your upper back touches the floor. Relax and feel the stretch.

Expert advice: The greatest stretch will be felt right above the wide sling. Move the wide sling farther up or down the back to target different parts of the back. This allows you to stretch any specific part of the spine you feel is tight.

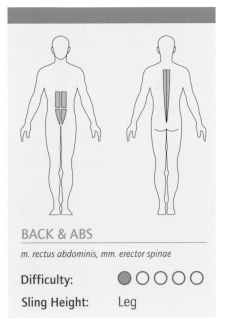

BACK & ABS

m. rectus abdominis, mm. erector spinae

Difficulty: ●○○○○
Sling Height: Leg

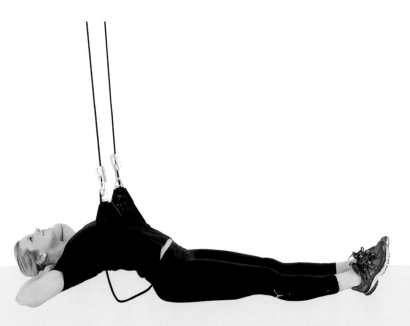

6.6   Pendulum

Lie on your back with your head in the wide sling. Relax and let the head rest. Move your head slowly left and right.

Expert advice: Let your head rest heavy in the sling. Feel the muscles of your neck. Try to release any tension by consciously relaxing your muscles. Feel your neck relaxing and the tension melt away.

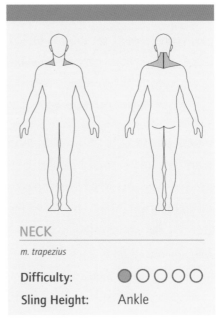

NECK

m. trapezius

Difficulty: ●○○○○

Sling Height: Ankle

137

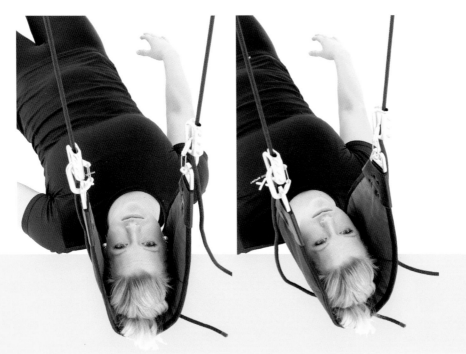

6.7 Sling splits

Place one leg in the sling in front of you. Lean forward on a straight leg, keeping your foot pointed forward. Feel a stretch in the hamstrings, the back of the thigh.

Expert advice: This is the definitive hamstring stretch used by ballet dancers and gymnasts. The farther up your leg you place the sling, the lower the force on the stretch. Begin with the sling up above your knee for a soft stretch and then adjust accordingly. If you feel a prickling sensation down lower leg or foot, you are stretching the nerve. Bend your knee slightly and keep your foot flexed upward.

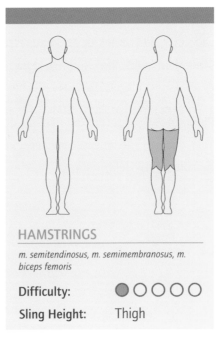

HAMSTRINGS

m. semitendinosus, m. semimembranosus, m. biceps femoris

Difficulty: ●○○○○

Sling Height: Thigh

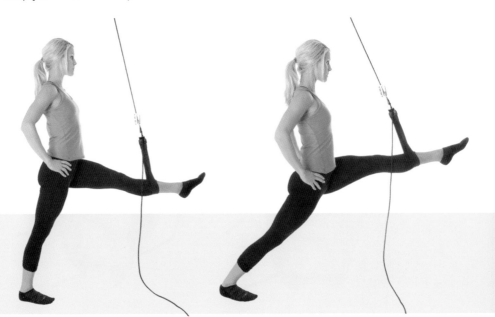

6.8 Hip rotators (Internal rotation hips)

Place one foot in the sling in front of you, letting the knee point out to the side. Hold on to the sling for balance and lean forward. You should feel a stretch through the outside of the thigh.

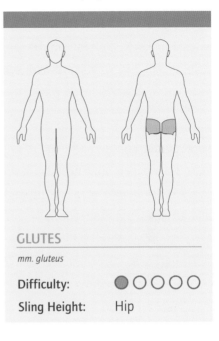

GLUTES

mm. gluteus

Difficulty: ●○○○○

Sling Height: Hip

139

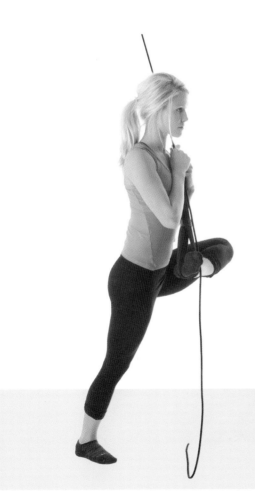

6.9 Hamstring stretch

Lie on your back and attach a free sling to one foot. With the leg straight, pull the sling and your leg toward you. Hold for 30 seconds before you let up.

Expert advice: You should feel the stretch in the back of your thigh. If you start feeling pins and needles down your leg, try flexing your foot upward and bending your knee slightly.

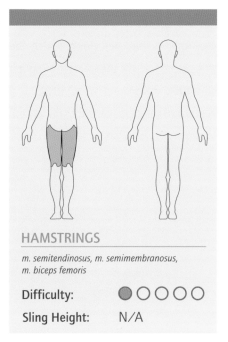

HAMSTRINGS

m. semitendinosus, m. semimembranosus, m. biceps femoris

Difficulty: ●○○○○

Sling Height: N/A

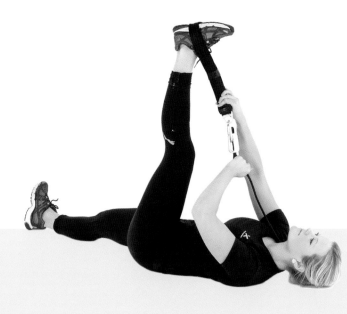

6.10 Glute stretch

Lie on your back and attach the sling to one foot. Bend your knee and pull the sling toward the opposite shoulder. Pull the foot toward you until you feel a stretch in the upper, outer thigh area. Hold for 30 seconds and then repeat with the opposite leg.

Expert advice: While pulling the leg toward you, support your knee with the free arm.

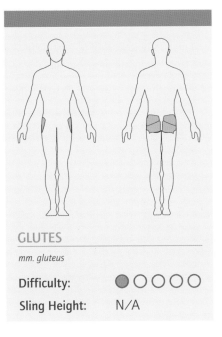

GLUTES

mm. gluteus

Difficulty: ●○○○○

Sling Height: N/A

141

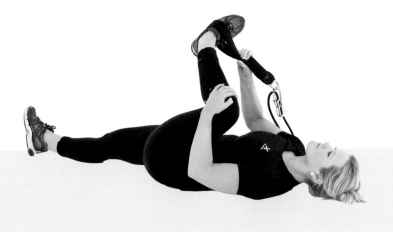

6.11   Quad stretch

With one leg bent backward, place the foot in the sling behind you. Tighten the loop (if applicable) to get a tight fit for your foot. Hold on to the sling for balance, lean back and push your hips forward. Feel the stretch in the quadriceps, the muscles of the front of the thigh.

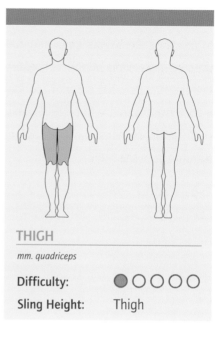

THIGH

mm. quadriceps

Difficulty: ●○○○○
Sling Height: Thigh

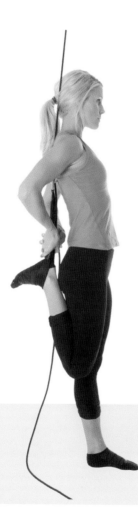

6.12 Hip flexor stretch

With one leg bent backward, place the foot in the sling behind you. Jump forward past the sling attachment point. Let the back leg stretch backward and gradually put your weight onto it. Keep your back in a neutral position and feel the stretch in the front of the hip.

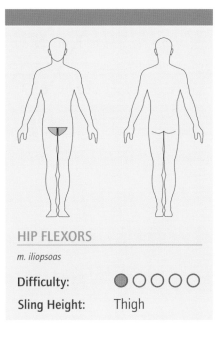

HIP FLEXORS

m. iliopsoas

Difficulty: ●○○○○

Sling Height: Thigh

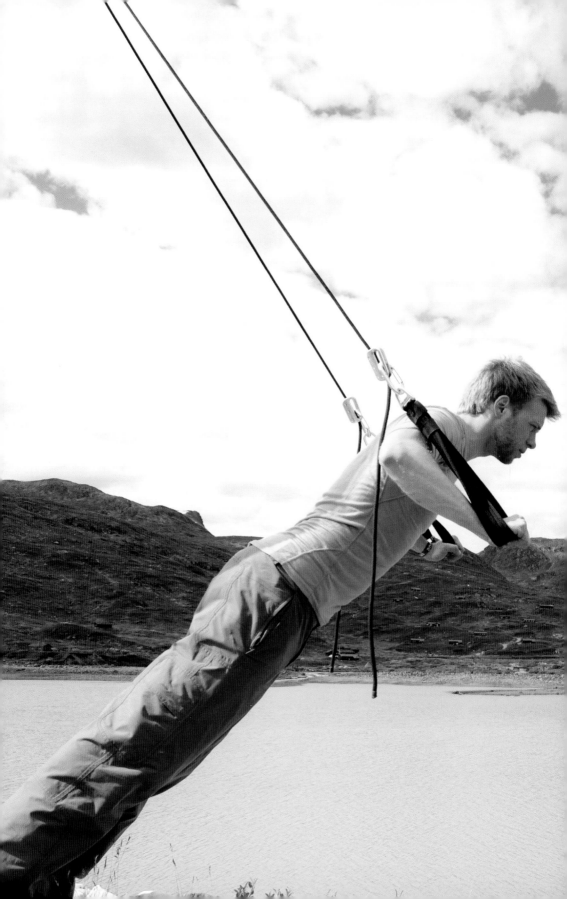

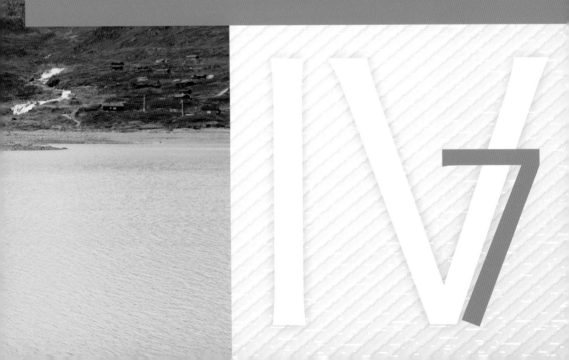

PART **IV**

CHAPTER 7

EXERCISES
SPORT SPECIFIC PROGRAMS

IV

7

Chapter 7

SPORT SPECIFIC PROGRAMS

SWIMMING   148

SNOWBOARDING   152

RUNNING   156

CLIMBING   160

VOLLEYBALL   164

TAEKWONDO   168

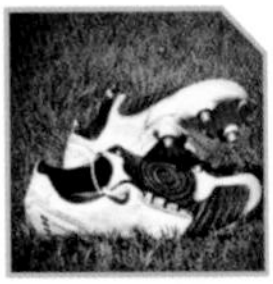

SOCCER   172

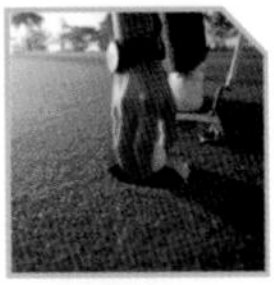

GOLF   176

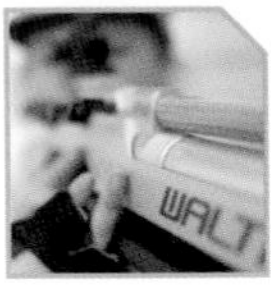

SHOOTING   180

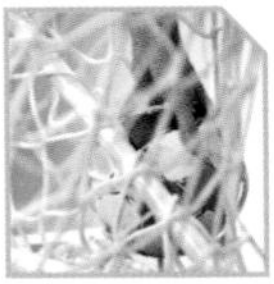

HANDBALL   184

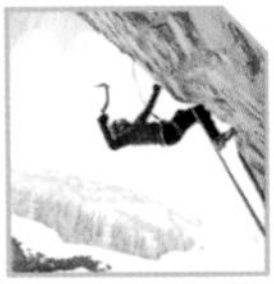

ICE CLIMBING   188

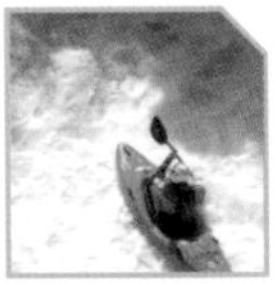

KAYAKING   192

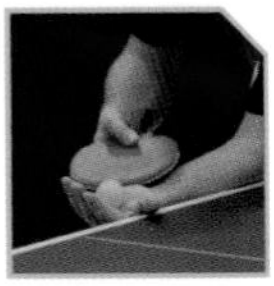

TABLE TENNIS   196

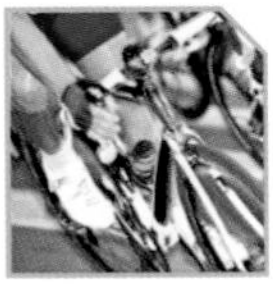

CYCLING   200

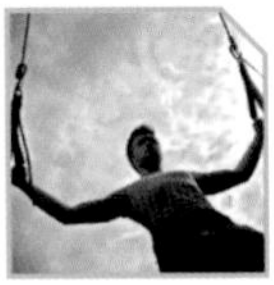

BASIC WORKOUTS   204

Sling training for swimming

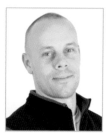

Name:	Terje Nitter
Education:	Physiotherapist HIB.
Occupation	
and experience:	Physical Therapist at Tonus Physiotherapy and Fitness. Course instructor for The Norwegian Olympic Sports Center. Many years of experience as a sling training course instructor.

> *We've used sling training since 2003 in our daily workouts, and we are seeing superb results. Slings offer infinite possibilities. We use them for our athletes at all levels, for prehab and performance development.*
>
> **Stig Leganger-Hansen**
>
> Coach for the Norwegian West Coast swim team and former coach for Alexander Dale Oen for 10 years

Reverse flies

see page 69

The plank

see page 92

Twisted plank

see page 96

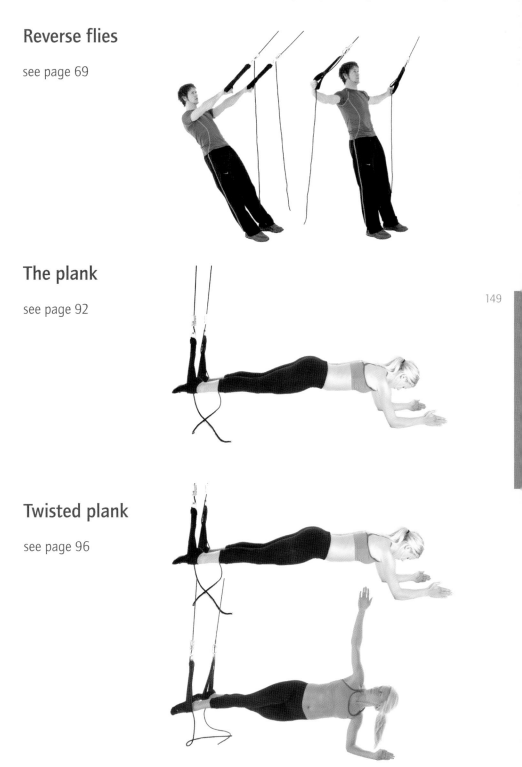

Hanging leg raises

see page 120

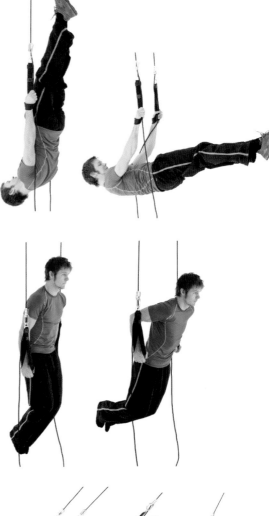

Dips

see page 85

Reverse flies
(slings crossed)

see page 69

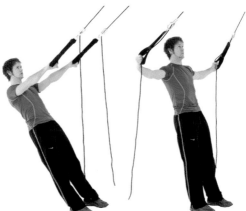

Two specific swimming exercises

Equipment needed: two sets of slings spaced nine feet (3 m) apart.

Both exercises start from the same position. For Example 1 Breaststroke do the movements from photos one and two. For Example 2 Keystroke, do the movements from photos one to three. Go for three sets of 6-8 reps.

Example 1 Breaststroke

Place a wide sling as far up on your thighs as possible. Adjust the other set of slings to a height of four feet (1.5 m). Grab the slings in front of you and lean forward until your feet are off the ground. Pull your hands down and out toward the sides in a broad stroke. Return slowly to starting position.

151

Example 2 Keystroke

Place a wide sling as far up on your thighs as possible. Adjust the other set of slings to a height of three feet (1 m). Grab the slings in front of you and lean forward until your feet are off the ground. Pull your hands down and out toward the sides in a broad stroke. Continue by pulling the hands in towards your midline and down to your thighs. Return slowly to starting position.

Expert advice: Adjust the difficulty by changing the height of the slings in front of you. Placing the wide sling lower (toward your knees) makes it more challenging for your core muscles.

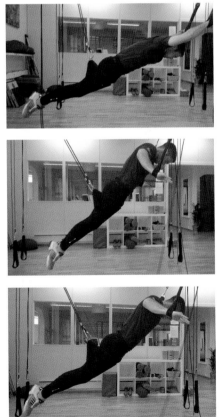

SNOWBOARDING

Sling training for snowboarding

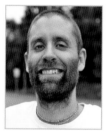

Name: Ole Christian Petterson

Occupation and experience: Marketing and photo editor at Playboard Magazine. Long-time skater and snowboarder

Super effective workout for functional strength. Agility and strength that suits boardsports!

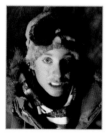

Name: Fredrik Austbø

Occupation and experience: Professional snowboarder and skater around the world

Instability exercise is a key to high performance. Sling training is great; it's versatile and makes you strong but not bulky.

Sprinter start

see page 46

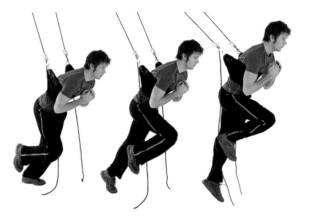

Backward lunge

see page 52

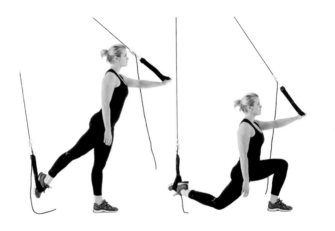

Backward lunge to jump

see page 53

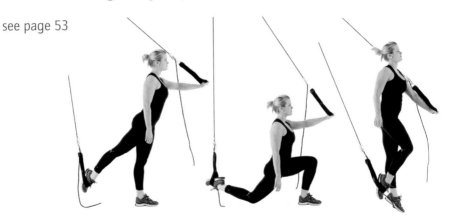

One leg deep squat

see page 55

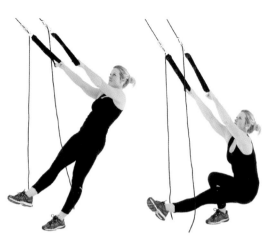

One leg hamstring curl

see page 58

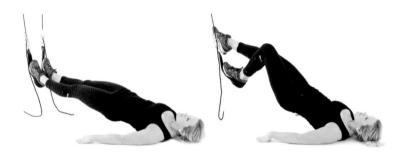

Push ups on a fitness ball

see page 83

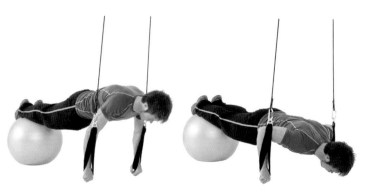

Twisted side plank

see page 113

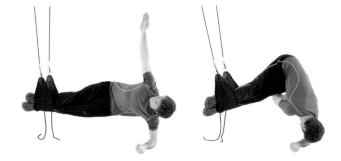

Sling squat

see page 127

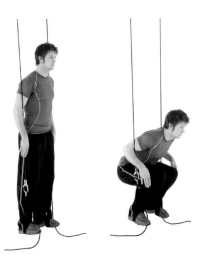

Expert advice: Do three sets of 12 reps.

Snowboarding and sling training: All the exercises from chapter 4 are recommended. A strong core is so important when it comes to drops and falls and preventing injuries. Snowboarders want agility and core strength. Too much muscle makes you slow and heavy. Become like Bruce Lee, not Arnold Schwarzenegger. If your workouts become easy, challenge your instability instead of adding weights.

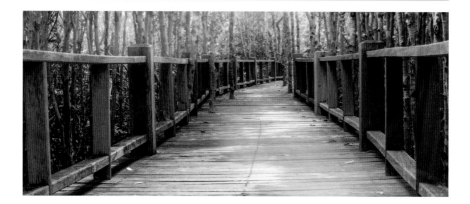

RUNNING

Sling training for running

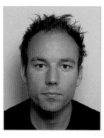

Name: John Henry Strupstad

Occupation and experience: Editor at Fysioterapeuten Magazine, winner of Oslo Marathon 2009, currently ultrarunner and Norwegian record holder for 50K runs

Many medium and long distance runners forget strength and mobility training. Maybe because they find it boring? Slings are a motivational, functional and efficient tool to target your core running muscles. Good luck!

Stability lunge

see page 54

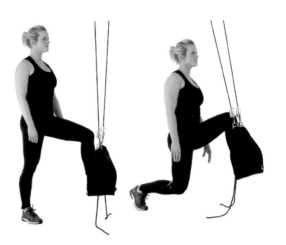

One leg deep squat

see page 55

If you are a medium- or long-distance runner, be careful about doing deep squats. This may build a disproportionate amount of muscle mass. Bending your knee to 90 degrees is sufficient.

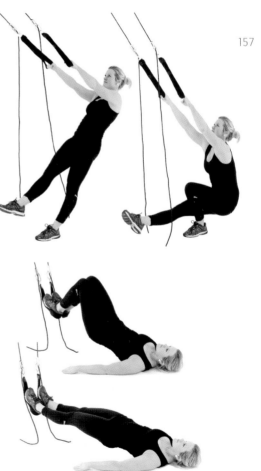

Hamstring curl

see page 56

Most runners are radically weaker in their hamstrings and glutes compared to the front of the thighs. These exercises will help to compensate for the asymmetry and improve your running economy.

One leg hamstring curl

see page 58

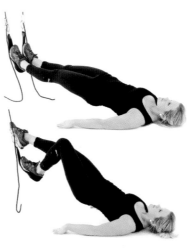

Sling cycling

see page 93

Omega

see page 94

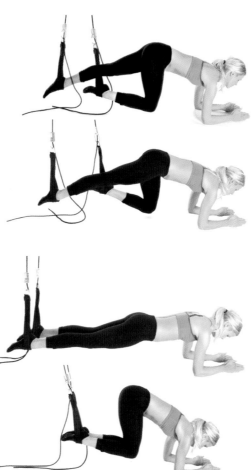

Sideways omega

see page 95

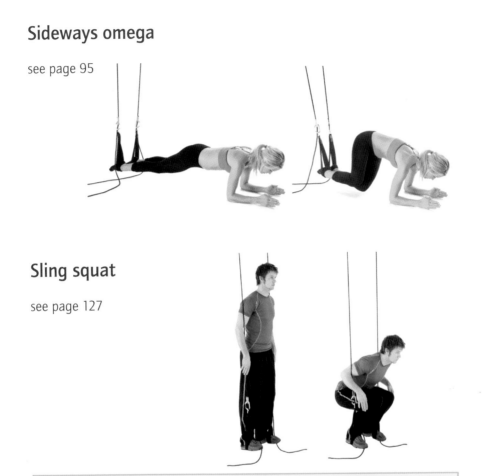

Sling squat

see page 127

Expert advice: Do three sets of 10 reps. Except core exercises Sling cycling, Omega and Sideways omega: Do these until failure to maintain perfect form.

Running and sling training: To become a good runner, you need to run. A lot. The strength workout should be quick but effective. These exercises are recommended right after a light run, 2-3 times a week.

This workout is meant as a supplement: The exercises will strengthen your running muscles and improve your running efficiency. These sling training exercises are well suited for athletes from 800 meters and up to marathon running.

Sling training for climbing

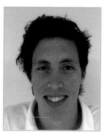

Name:	Stian Christophersen
Occupation	
and experience:	Norwegian bouldering champion 2009, Physical therapist at Nydalen Fysio, National team coach for the Norwegian Climbing Association

After I added sling training to my routine, my shoulder problems were eliminated. Sling training increases core strength and has meant a lot to me as a climber. Sling training injury-proofs your body: You can sustain more challenges without injuries if you add a weekly sling workout.

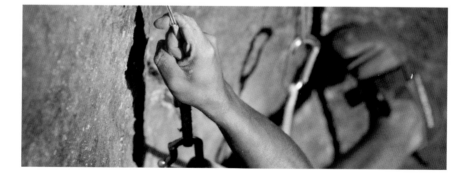

Superman

see page 65

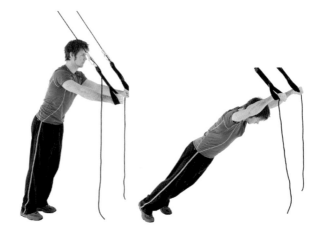

Superman/Flies

see page 65/67

161

Begin by doing the movements in Superman (exercise 3.2), but do not lean as far forward. Move the arms outwards and squeeze the shoulder blades, finishing off in the end position of flies (exercise 3.4). Return to starting position for Superman.

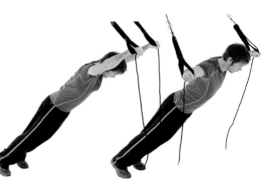

Internal rotation

see page 77

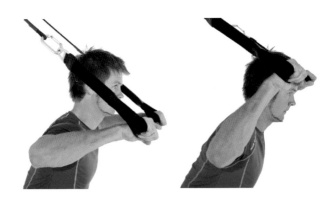

External rotation

see page 76

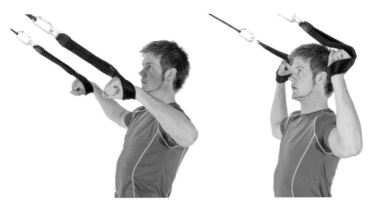

Incline pull-ups

see page 73

To increase difficulty, try these with your legs on a ball or bench.

Push-ups on a fitness ball

see page 83

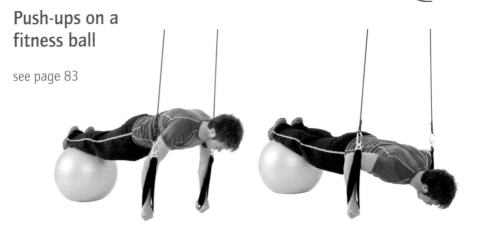

Omega

see page 94

Try this one with the right knee touching the left elbow and vice versa, as in exercise 4.6 Sideways omega.

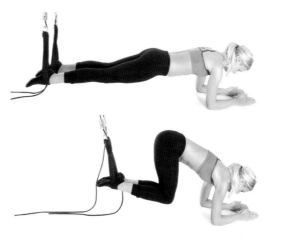

Incline handstand press

see page 111

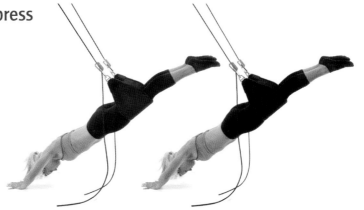

Expert advice: The exercises should be strenuous, do two sets of 5-8 reps twice a week.

Sling training for volleyball

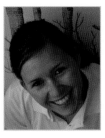

Name: Maria Øgreid Leitao

Occupation
and experience: Physical therapist at Stavanger Sports
Clinic, Physical therapist on FIVB World
Tour

After I began doing sling training I am stronger, more agile and
have had less injuries. I now use the slings both as a workout and
as a warm-up every day before hitting the sand.

Tarjei Skarlund
Professional beach volleyball player

High hamstring curl

see page 57

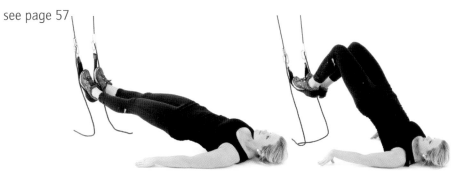

Superman

see page 65

165

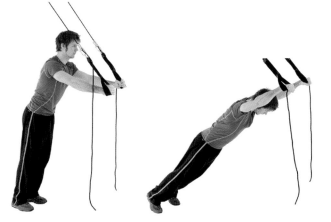

Push-ups

see page 83

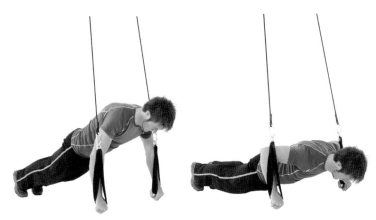

Pull-ups

see page 86

Omega

see page 94

Sling squat

see page 127

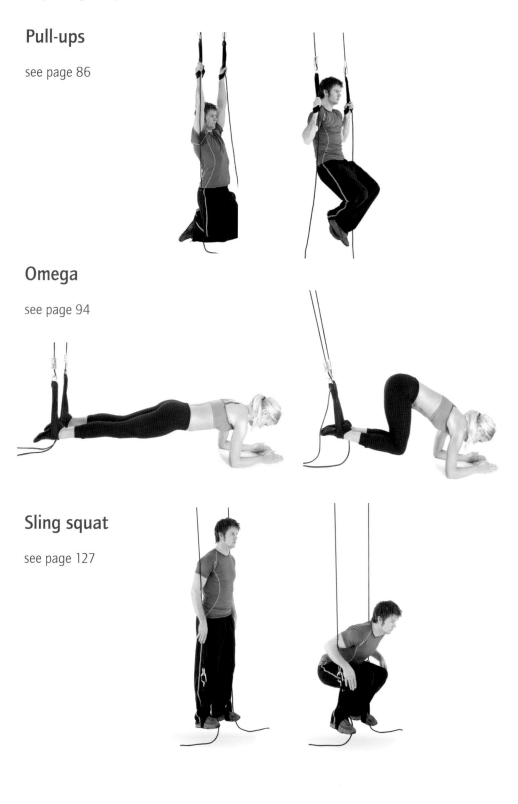

Specific volleyball exercise: Back extension to smash

Begin with a wide sling at your hips. Lean forward, and have a partner hold your legs to find the balance lying in the sling. Lift your upper body from the floor before imitating the smash movement. Use the opposite arm to guide the direction of the smash. Repeat for other arm.

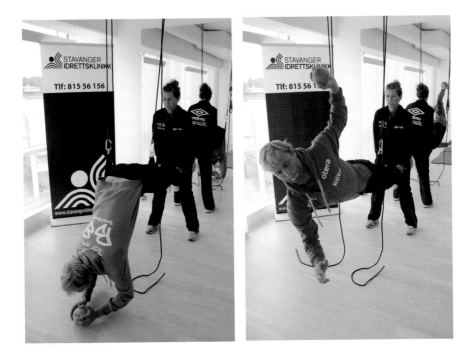

Expert advice: Do three sets of 4-6 reps. Adjust the exercises to suit your level. We've found that sport performance increases by performing these exercises. For example, a harder and more precise smash in the field.

TAEKWONDO

Sling training for taekwondo

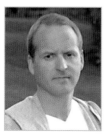

Name: Vegard Iversen

Occupation and experience: Associate professor at the sports section of Bergen College, Coach for the national team of the International Taekwondo Federation

For me, in taekwondo, it is paramount to be strong throughout the body. Training in slings, I have increased my strength and technique while keeping injuries away.

Marielle Lind

World cup winner 2012, European champion 2012 and 2011

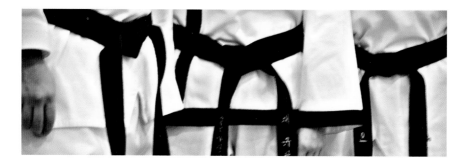

One leg hamstring curl

see page 58

If this one is too easy for you, move on to 5.17 The egg.

Superman

see page 65

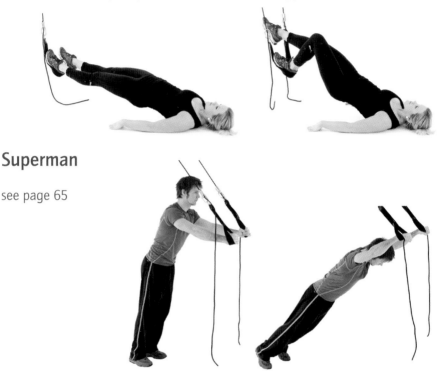

Incline pull-ups

see page 73

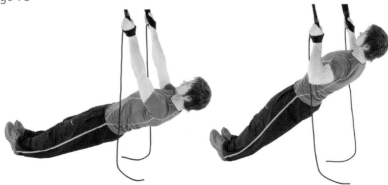

Push-ups

see page 83

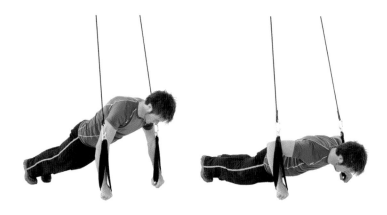

Omega

see page 94

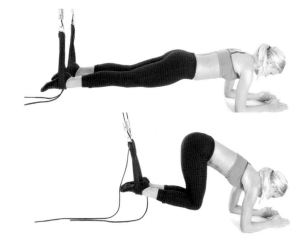

Dynamic side plank

see page 100

You may combine this one with exercise 2.11 Sling leg lifts and 2.12 Inner thigh lifts to increase load on the thigh muscles.

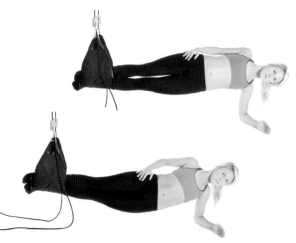

Sling squat

see page 127

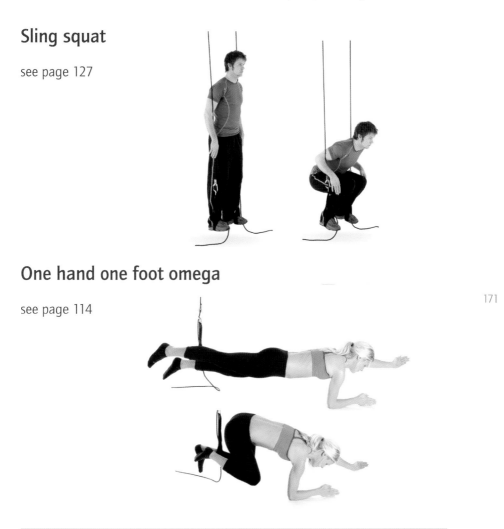

One hand one foot omega

see page 114

Expert advice: Do three sets of 6-8 reps for all exercises.

Taekwondo and sling training: Taekwondo is a sport that requires great balance, strength and mobility. Sling training may help to prevent injuries. Therefore, we've added slings to our exercise programs.

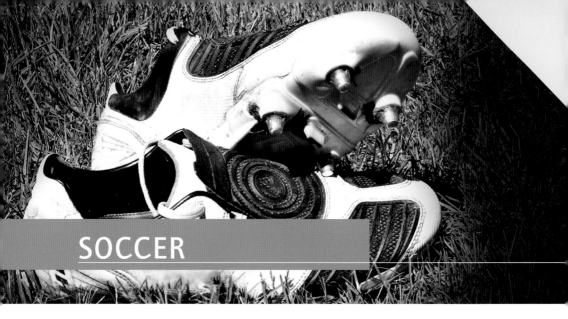

SOCCER

Sling training for soccer

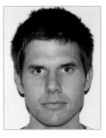

Name: Halvard Grova

Occupation and experience: Msc. Physical therapist with speciali-zation in sports, physical therapist for Viking Football Club

Sling training is an excellent way to train functional strength. It is one of my most important tools when working with athletes.

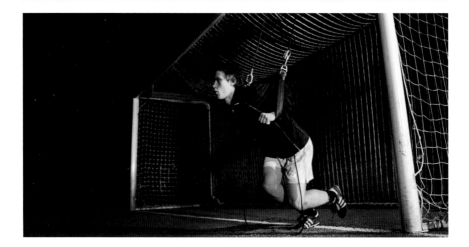

Backward lunge

see page 52

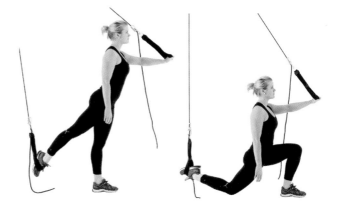

High hamstring curl

see page 57

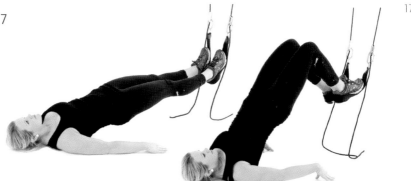

Sling leg lifts

see page 60

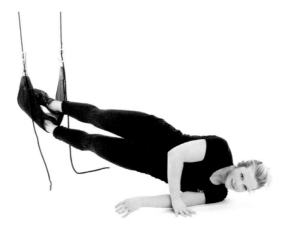

Inner thigh lifts

see page 61

Hold the end position for 10 seconds. Then do 10 controlled repetitions without pause.

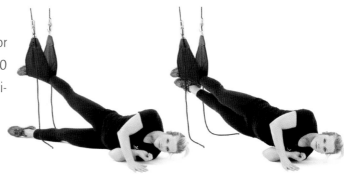

The plank

see page 92

Try this variation: Have one foot in the sling, and lift the free foot toward the ceiling. Pretend that you are kicking backward. Repeat 10 times.

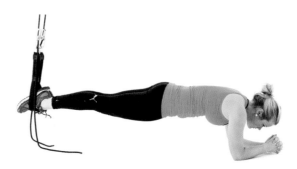

Supine plank rotation

see page 103

Hold the starting position for 10 seconds before doing 10 reps.

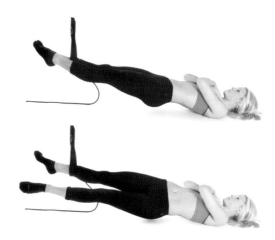

One hand one foot omega

see page 114

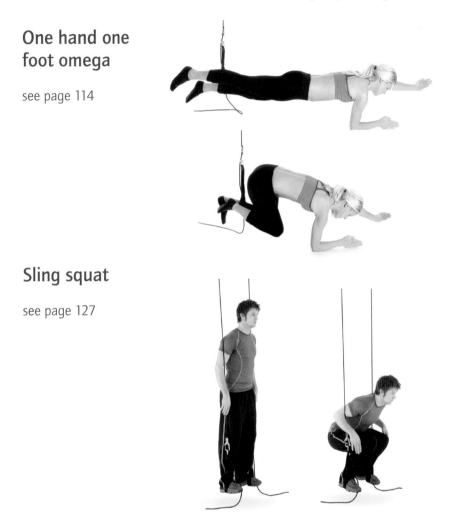

Sling squat

see page 127

Expert advice: Do three sets of 10 reps each. For the plank, hold for 30-60 seconds.

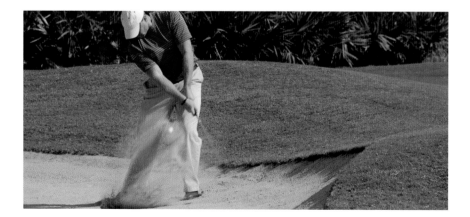

GOLF

Sling training for golfing

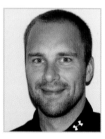

Name: Marcus Petterson

**Occupation
and experience:**   Physical therapist and personal trainer,
                    Sportsphysio for golfers on the Euro-
                    pean Tour, CEO of Betterperformance

*I implement slings in golf training because of the opportunity for
many specific movements. The athletes stay injury-free and get
motivated to train functionally and specifically.*

Sling leg lifts

see page 60

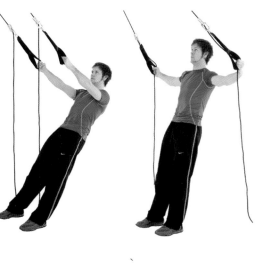

Reverse flies

see page 69

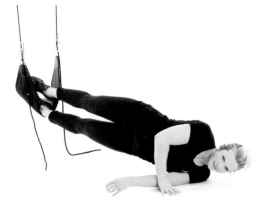

One arm row

see page 72

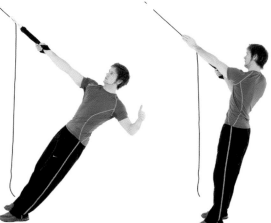

Omega

see page 94

Dynamic side plank

see page 100

Supine plank rotation

see page 103

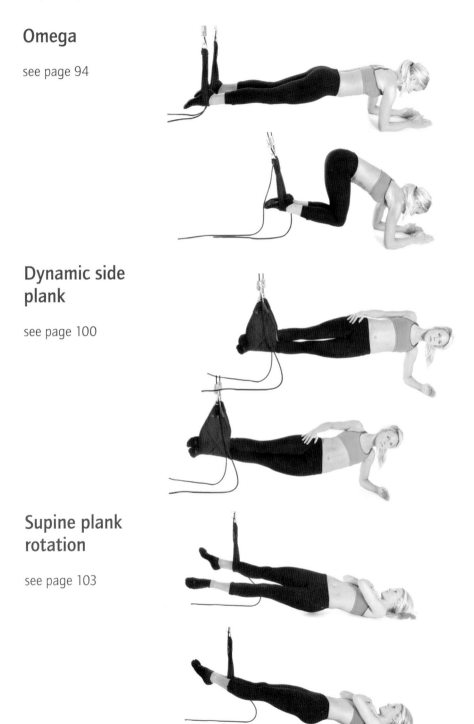

Specific exercise: Rotating cross

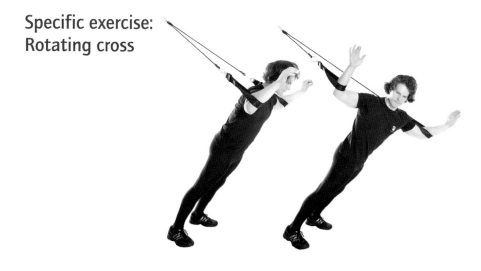

The movement begins in the end position of Flies (exercise 3.4), with the sling fastened around your forearms. Hold your hips steady and rotate your upper body slowly to one side. Return slowly and repeat to other side.

179

Expert advice: This holistic workout may be used throughout the golf season. Do four sets of 6-8 reps.

Golf and sling training: If you look at golfers today compared with the pre-Tiger Woods period, there is a whole new level of strength and consistency in the swing. Golfers need both explosive strength and endurance to maintain accuracy over long periods.

SHOOTING

Sling training for shooting

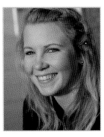

Name: Charlotte Taanevig

**Occupation
and experience:**   Physical therapist, Female Norwegian
rifle shooting champion 2010

*It has always been important for me to build and maintain strong
core muscles to keep the best firing position.*

Espen Berg-Knutsen

Norwegian, European and World rifle shooting champion

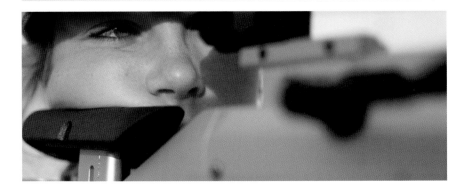

Superman

see page 65

Incline pull-ups

see page 73

Side press

see page 75

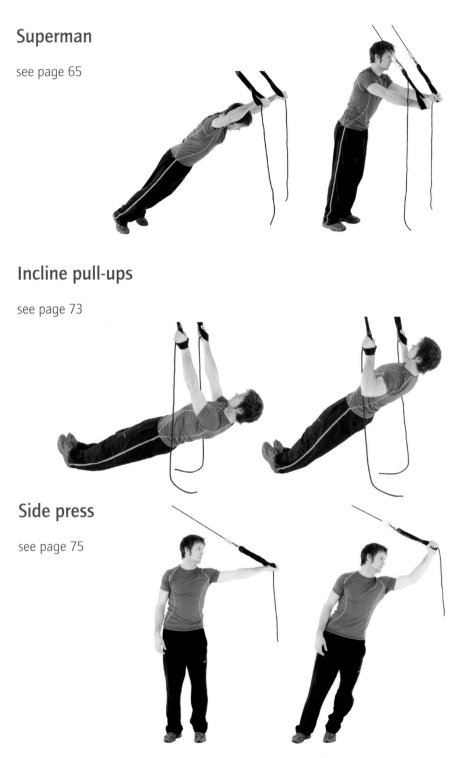

The plank

see page 92

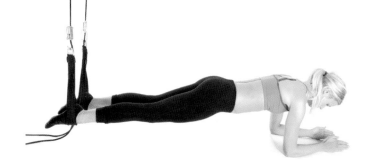

Twisted plank

see page 96

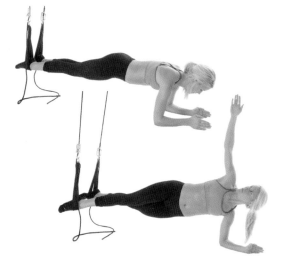

Delta

see page 97

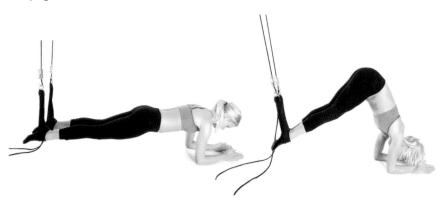

Side plank

see page 99

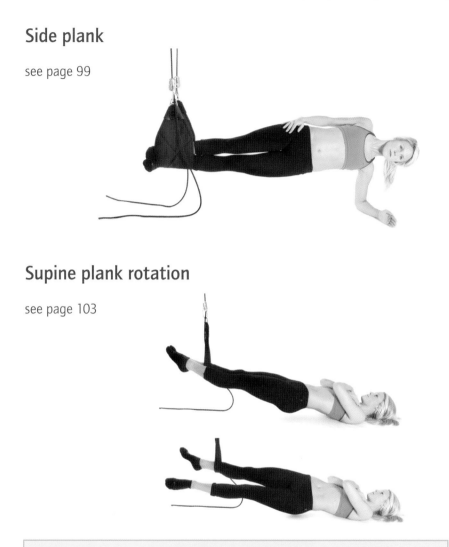

Supine plank rotation

see page 103

183

Expert advice: To make this workout highly relevant for the sport of shooting, you should aim for many sets (3-8) and many repetitions (15-20) with short breaks (30 sec-1 min).

Shooting and sling training: Shooting is a static sport where you lie down, sit or stand in the same position for a long time. This creates asymmetrical strain on the tissues of the body. Strengthening and stabilizing the core may help to prevent sports injuries.

HANDBALL

Sling training for handball

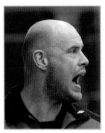

Name: Mika Nurmi

Occupation and experience: Coach for Haugaland Handballclub, Lecturer at the handball section of Haugesund Elite Sports Academy

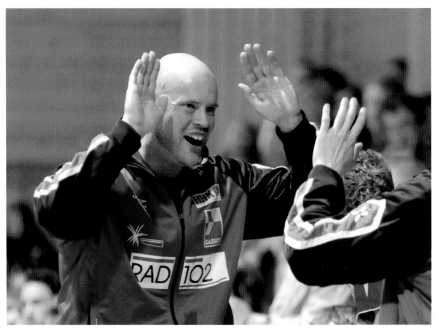

Postural squat

see page 47

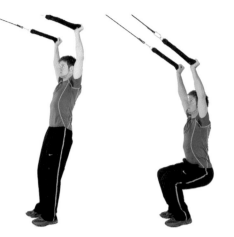

Backward lunge

see page 52

Stability lunge

see page 54

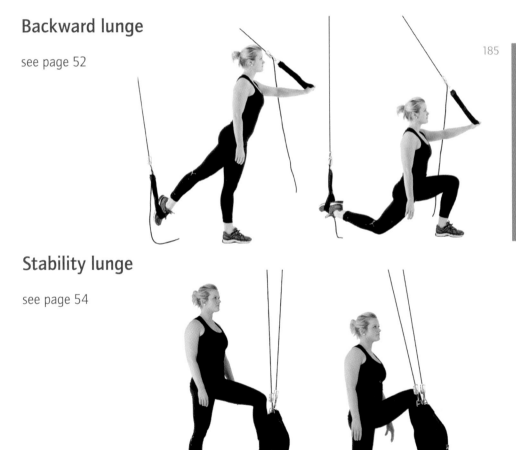

Supported dips

see page 84

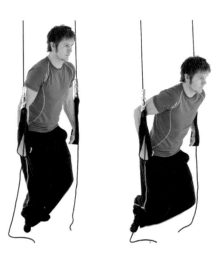

The plank

see page 92

Supine plank

see page 101

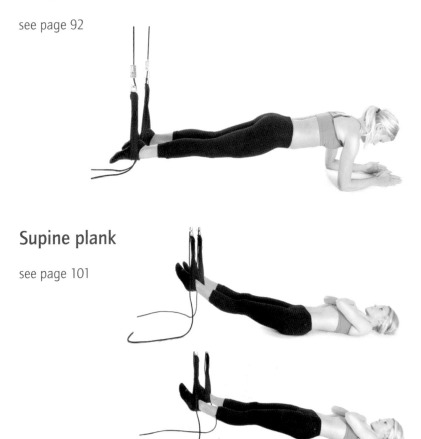

Incline handstand press

see page 111

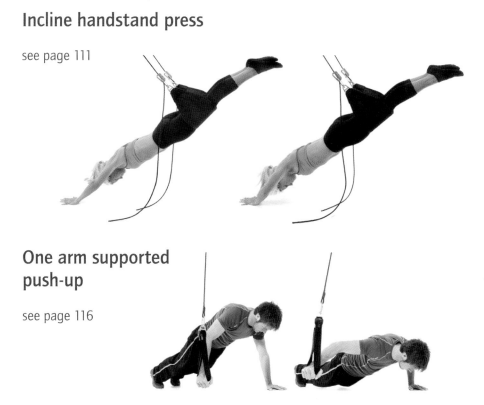

One arm supported push-up

187

see page 116

Expert advice: Do three sets of 4-6 repetitions.

Handball and sling training: During the season, athletes need to perform at their best in every game. Sling training is a valuable supplement to our workouts to create and maintain high performance for prolonged periods.

ICE CLIMBING

Sling training for ice climbing

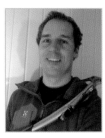

Name: Erik Mowinckel

Occupation

and experience: Physical therapist and ice climber, pre-
viously coach for snowboarders and
climbers

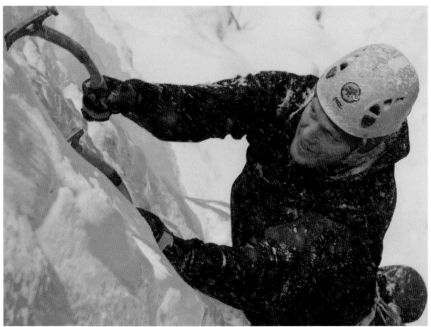

Postural squat

see page 47

Flies

see page 67

Reverse flies

see page 69

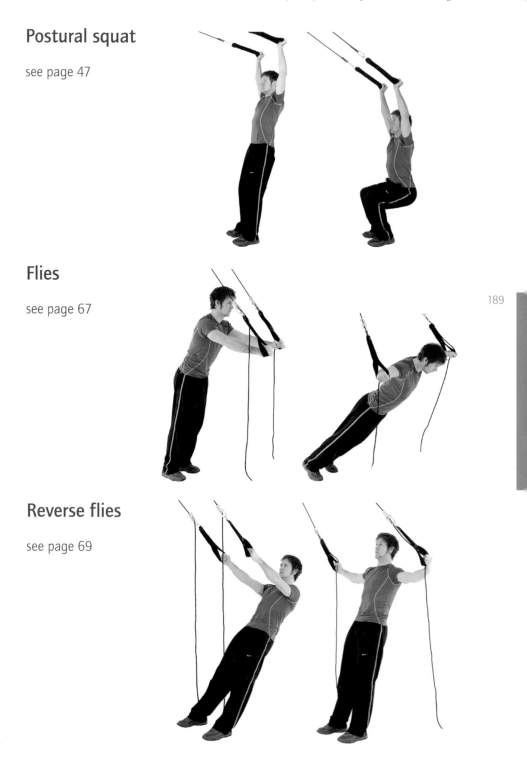

One arm row

see page 72

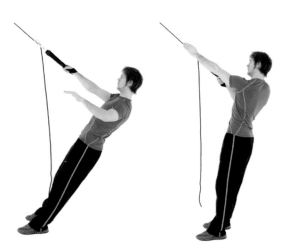

Side press

see page 75

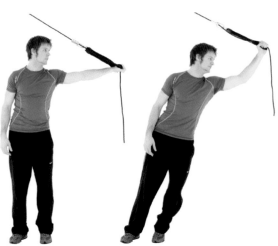

Sideways omega

see page 95

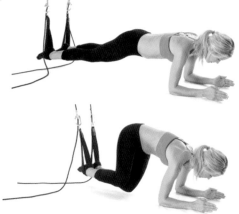

Specific exercise:
Figure 4 / 9

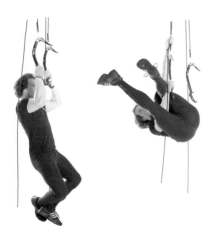

Hang on to the slings, or preferably on to axes, with straight arms. Lift your legs and cross the left leg over the right arm. Try to get your leg up as far as possible.

Pull your chest up, let go of the left hand and reach up over the right hand as high as you can. Hold this position for 3-4 seconds, then return slowly all the way down and repeat to opposite side.

Expert advice: Hold the slings like you would hold the shaft of the ice axe. If possible, hook the axe directly onto the carabiner and hold on to the shaft.

Use a small step box or something similar and stand on your toes with your heels low. This imitates the way you would stand to keep your grip on the ice.

Ice climbing and sling training: Ice climbing is mostly repeating a few identical movements. The ice conditions, quality and steepness will affect the degree of core stability you need to hang on. Bad footholds demand more upper body strength and stability. Mixed climbing on ice and rock provides more technical challenges.

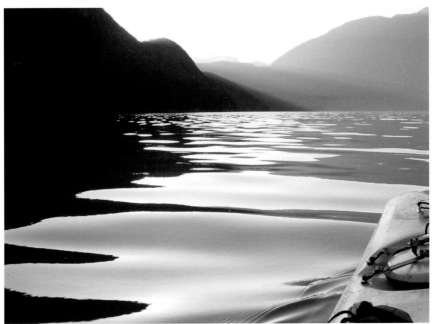

KAYAKING

Sling training for kayaking

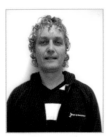

Name: Marius Holst Meinseth

**Occupation
and Experience:**   Physical therapist, physical therapist
for the Norwegian rowing and kaya-
king Olympic and world championship
teams

Incline pull-ups

see page 73

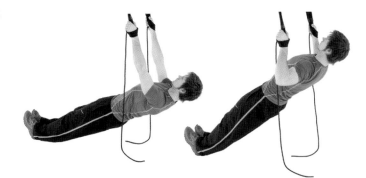

Push-ups

see page 83

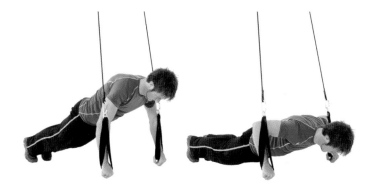

Dips

see page 85

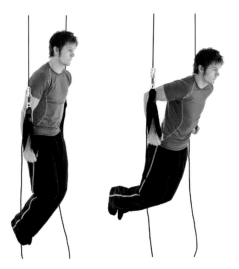

The plank

see page 92

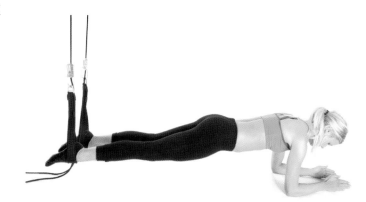

Leg lifts

see page 106

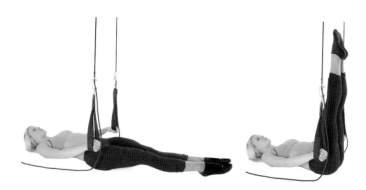

Handstand Press

see page 112

Walk in wheelbarrow motion from push-up position to handstand and back down.

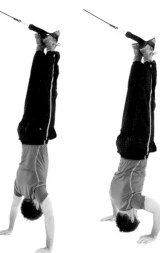

Expert advice:

This workout is designed to make you a better kayaker by strengthening your sport specific muscles. Do four sets of 8-12 repetitions. To make the workout more challenging, add instability.

Kayaking and sling training: If you want to be a better kayaker, you need core, upper body rotation and shoulder area strength. The exercises provided here are often used in pre-season training. Adjust the difficulty and number of reps to suit your capabilities.

Sling training for table tennis

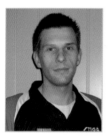

Name: Joachim Sørensen

Occupation

and experience: Physical and manual therapist, Medical advisor for the Norwegian Table Tennis Federation, Sportsphysio in the Paralympics

> *Sling training is a valuable tool for table tennis players. It's useful for building basic and explosive strength.*

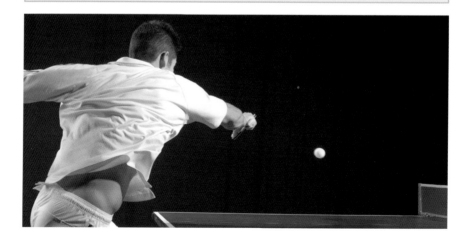

External rotation

see page 76

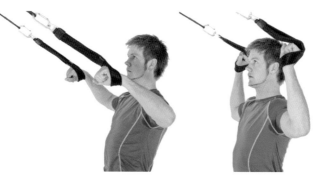

Internal rotation

see page 77

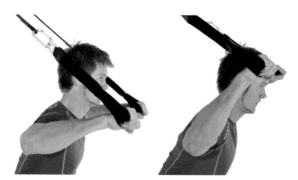

Push-ups on a fitness ball

see page 83

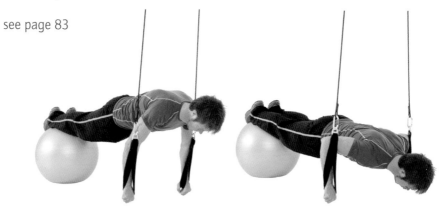

Supine plank rotation

see page 103

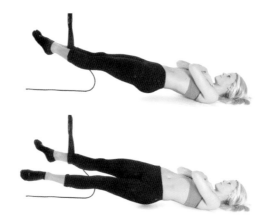

Twisted side plank

see page 113

Sling squat

see page 127

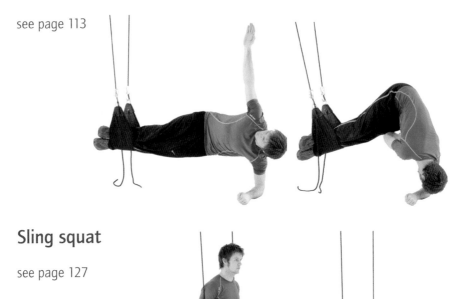

Specific exercise: Rotating cross

see page 179

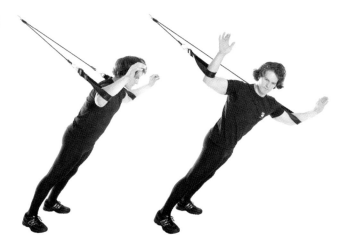

Expert advice: Do three sets of 4-6 repetitions.

Table tennis and sling training: Table tennis is a sport where you stop and go constantly in short rallies. Your focus in strength training should be on maximum strength at maximum speed to build explosive strength.

You should also add some stretching from chapter 6 at the end of your workouts to maintain and increase mobility in the upper back and shoulders.

CYCLING

Sling training for cycling

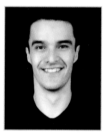

Name: Frank Rizzo

Occupation and experience: Physical therapist, Physical trainer for football, cycling and running teams, CEO of Betterperformance.

The strong core muscles I've developed through sling training let me supply more power to the pedals while also improving my running economy.

Jonathan Love

Hawaiian Ironman World Championship contestant

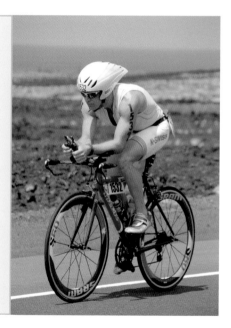

Postural squat

see page 47

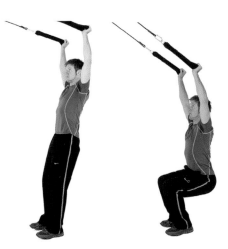

One leg hamstring curl

see page 58

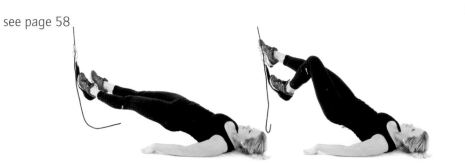

High extension to splits

see page 59

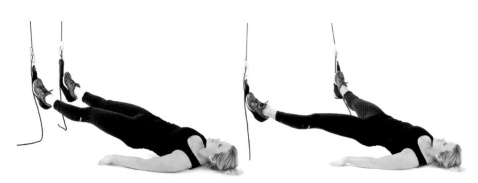

Incline pull-ups

see page 82

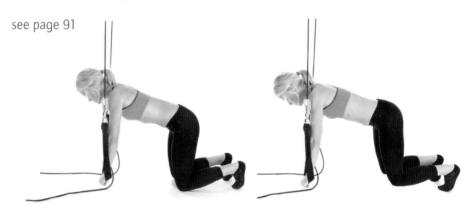

Knees off the ground

see page 91

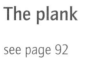

The plank

see page 92

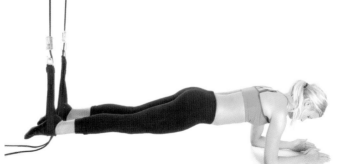

Sling cycling

see page 93

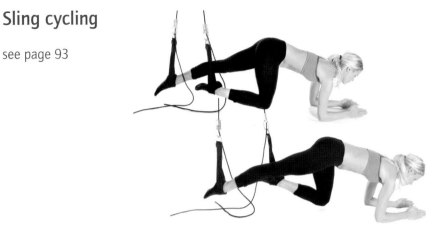

One leg supine plank

see page 102

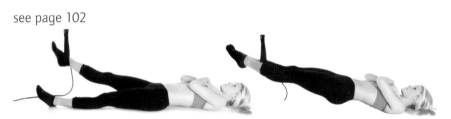

Expert advice: This holistic workout may be used throughout the cycling season. Do four sets of 6-8 reps.

Cycling and sling training: A new study[1] shows the relationship between the biomechanics of cycling and core muscle strength. Weak core muscles and lack of core stability may add strain on the knee joint, which can lead to injuries.

Beginning cyclists often lack the basic core strength. Ideally, cyclists should begin core training when they first start cycling. Sling training strengthens your core muscles, specifically around the hips, and this increases performance and keeps you injury-free.

1   Smogila, JM et al. (2007). Relationship between cycling mechanics and core stability. *J Strength Cond Res.*, *21*(4), 1300-4.

BASIC WORKOUTS

Beginner program 30 min

Warm-up (10 min)

- ▶ 1.1   Squat and row (whole body)
- ▶ 1.2   Lunge and fly (whole body)

Strength exercises (20 min)

15 reps x 3 sets

- ▶ 3.19 Incline push-ups
- ▶ 3.5   Reverse elbow flies
- ▶ 2.1   One leg squat
- ▶ 3.10 Incline pull-ups
- ▶ 4.3   The plank
- ▶ 2.7   Hamstring curl
- ▶ 3.15 Hammer curls
- ▶ 3.17 Triceps press

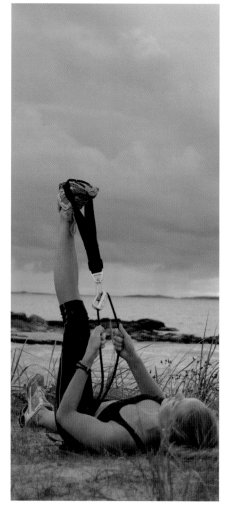

Express program 20 min
Upper body/core

5–7 reps x 2 sets – two and two exercises are performed in pairs. Do two sets before you continue to the next two exercises.

Example: Flies – Reverse flies – Flies –Reverse flies – Push-ups – etc.

Warm-up (10 min)
- ▶ 1.1 Squat and row
- ▶ 1.2 Lunge and fly

Strength exercises
- ▶ 3.4 Flies
- ▶ 3.6 Reverse flies
- ▶ 3.13 External rotation
- ▶ 3.10 Incline pull-ups
- ▶ 3.20 Push-ups in combination with
- ▶ 4.5 Omega
- ▶ 4.11 Dynamic side plank
- ▶ 3.24 Pull-ups
- ▶ 3.18 One arm triceps press

205

Express program 20 min
Core/thighs

5–7 reps x 2 sets – two and two exercises are performed in pairs. Do two sets before you continue to the next two exercises.

Example: Omega – High hamstring curl – Omega – High hamstring curl – Backward lunge - etc.

Warm-up (10 min)

- ▶ 1.1 Squat and row
- ▶ 1.3 Lunge with side bend
- ▶ 4.5 Omega
- ▶ 2.8 High hamstring curl
- ▶ 2.3 Backward lunge
- ▶ 2.11 Sling leg lifts
- ▶ 4.17 Leg lifts
- ▶ 4.10 Side plank
- ▶ 3.15 Hammer curls
- ▶ 3.17 Triceps press

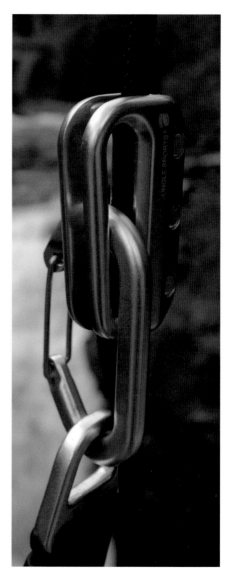

EXTREME program

6 reps x 3 sets – two and two exercises are performed in pairs. Do two sets before you continue to the next two exercises.

Example: Backward lunge to jump – High hamstring curl – Backward lunge to jump – High hamstring curl – Twisted side plank – etc.

Free warm-up 10 min

Strength exercises

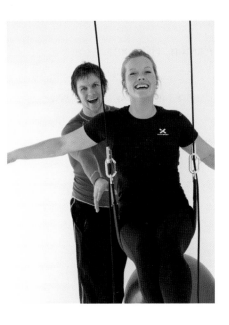

- ▶ 2.4 Backward lunge to jump
- ▶ 2.8 High hamstring curl
- ▶ 4.8 Delta in combination with
- ▶ 4.9 Body saw
- ▶ 5.4 Twisted side plank
- ▶ 5.16 Twisted push-ups
- ▶ 3.7 Y-flies
- ▶ 5.3 Handstand press
- ▶ 5.13 V-ups
- ▶ 5.20 Typewriter pull-ups
- ▶ 3.23 Dips

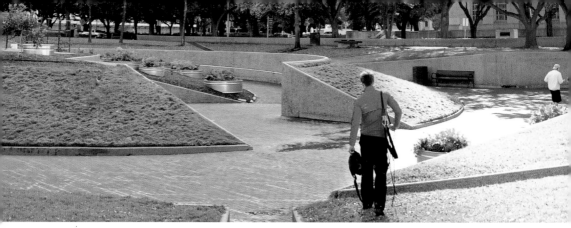

Credits

▶ iStockphoto/Thinkstock (p. 156 bottom, p. 160 bottom, p. 184 header, p. 192 bottom)

▶ iStockphoto.com (p. 148 header, p. 168 both, p. 176 both, p. 177 both, p. 191 both, p. 196 header, p. 200 header)

▶ Ryan McVay/Lifesize/gettyimages.de/Thinkstock (p. 196 bottom)

▶ Tonus fysioterapi og trening (p. 151)

▶ Olav Stubberud (p. 152 header – model: Fredrik Austbø)

▶ Ian Hollows (p. 160)

▶ Maria Øgreid Leitao (p. 167)

▶ Jungle Sports AS (man in goal post p. 172)

▶ Anders Aasen Berget (p. 180 both, p. 204)

▶ Morten Johansen (p. 188 both)

▶ Kayak Voss (www.kayakvoss.com) (p. 191 header)

▶ Betterperformance (http://betterperformance.no) (p. 200)

▶ Lennart Krohn-Hansen (p. 206)

▶ Gry Thorsen (p. 207)

▶ Hoby Finn/Photodisc/Thinkstock (p. 156 header)

▶ Imago (p. 184)

▶ Hemera/Thinkstock (p. 164 header)

▶ All portrait photos in chapter 7 are taken from the athlete's personal archives.

▶ All other chapter pictures are taken either by Andres Aasen Berget or Lennart Krohn-Hansen

Typesetting and page layout: Cornelia Knorr

Cover design: Andrea Brücher

Copy editing: Elizabeth Evans